Preschool Children
with Special
Health Care Needs

Preschool Children with Special Health Care Needs

Mary Theresa Urbano, Ph.D., R.N., A.R.N.P.
University of Miami School of Medicine
Department of Pediatrics
Mailman Center for Child Development (UAP)
Miami, Florida

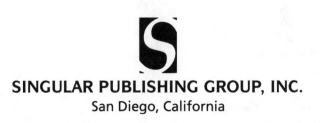

SINGULAR PUBLISHING GROUP, INC.
San Diego, California

Typeset by House Graphics
Typeset in 10/12 Palatino
Designed by Randy Stevens
Printed by McNaughton & Gunn

Art for figures 6-9, 6-10, 6-19, 6-21, and 6-22 by Teri A. Sherrin

Singular Publishing Group, Inc.
4284 41st Street
San Diego, California 92105-1197

Library of Congress Cataloging-in-Publication Data
Urbano, Mary Theresa.
    Preschool children with special health care needs / by Mary
Theresa Urbano.
        p.   cm.
    Includes index.
    ISBN 1-879105-41-1
    1. Preschool children—Diseases—Treatment. 2. Preschool
children—Health and hygiene.   I. Title.
    [DNLM: 1. Child Health Services—organization & administration.
2. Child, preschool—education. 3. Education, Special. 4. Family.
5. Handicapped.   6. Rehabilitation—in infancy & childhood.   WB320
U72p]
RJ47.U73   1991
618.92—dc20
DNLM/DLC
for Library of Congress   91-5140
                                                                             CIP

Printed in the United States of America

CONTENTS

of a Health-Related Procedure • Clean Intermittent Catheterization • Tube Feedings • Suctioning of the Nose and Mouth by Machine • Suctioning of the Nose Using Nasal Aspirator or Bulb Syringe • Tracheostomy Management • Suctioning the Tracheostomy • Using a Manual Resuscitator • Changing the Tracheostomy Tube • Changing the Tracheostomy Ties • Tracheostomy Skin Care • Oxygen Administration • Mechanical Ventilation

ACKNOWLEDGMENTS

I would like to thank the many friends, parents, and professional colleagues who contributed to the inspiration and development of this text. I am particularly grateful to the following individuals who provided invaluable reviews of specific content areas: Carole Abbott, Saribel Ceballos, Linda Friedman, Maria Gomez, Mirtha Gonzalez, Ileana Hernandez, Helen Masin, Ann-Britt Murphy, Raquel Rodriguez, Teri Sherrin, Michelle Sutton, and Lois Wilson. A special thank you to Anne Crane, Cathy Berkowitz, Pamela Tetlow, Jennifer Urbano, and Richard Urbano for their patience, support, encouragement, and input. I am also indebted to my steadfast friends, Keith and Marcia Scott, who are always there, no matter what. Thanks to Michael Bender of the Kennedy Institute, Johns Hopkins University, who served as the Consulting Editor for this manuscript. It was he who proposed the development of this text, and guided me through the exciting world of publishing. His leadership made the journey simple and hassle-free. Thanks also to Linton M. Vandiver and Marie Linvill from Singular Publishing Group for the opportunity to share my thoughts with others throughout the country and for their obvious commitment to quality. It is my hope that this text's contents will help to improve the quality of life for children with special health care needs and that of their families.

M.T.U.

This book is dedicated to Rick, for his love,
wisdom, and support through the years, and Jenni
for her love, assistance, and the gift of time

PREFACE

This text is about the health needs shared by all children: prevention of infections and accidents, monitoring of general growth and development, immunizations, appropriate food and liquids, adequate time for sleep and play, a stimulating environment, and nurturing and loving caregivers. However, it is primarily about ways to assist the child with special health care needs.

Follow this scenario, if you will.

The door opened, and the children scampered onto the playground, scrambling to be first on the swings or the slide. Jane Smith, their teacher, stood in the doorway, surveying the group of active toddlers. She smiled as she saw the children become absorbed with their activities. Each child had an individualized personality and unique abilities, yet they shared so much. It would have been impossible for the casual observer to be aware that Johnny, on the swings, would need a dose of his seizure medication soon. Or, that Maryanne, on the merry-go-round, would need to be catheterized shortly. Miss Smith was prepared to meet these special health care needs.

Not so long ago, Johnny and Maryanne would not have been a part of this group. They would have been cared for in a hospital or in their homes. Now, with changing technology and attitudes, increasing numbers of children with special health care needs are more fully integrated into their communities. With the changing emphasis to family centered, community-based care, health is becoming the concern of everyone working with children.

This text is designed to be a practical guide to professionals working in preschool settings. It addresses the continuum from basic primary health care important to all children, to management of complex medical conditions. Although some time is spent discussing specific conditions, the major focus is on the process of early identification and practical management of special health care needs of preschoolers. Knowledge of these basic concepts will assist the reader in developing competency in health-related areas important to all professionals. As a result, children with special health care needs will be able to participate in growth-enriching environments desired by all children and their families.

1

THE CHILD WITH SPECIAL HEALTH CARE NEEDS

E arly intervention is the challenge of the 1990s. It represents an exciting time for professionals interested in improving services for preschoolers and their families. The Education of the Handicapped Amendments of 1986 (P.L. 99-457) is scheduled to be implemented in the early 1990s. This legislation will expand diagnostic and intervention programs for many infants and children with, or at risk for, developmental disabilities. For the first time, there are major funding incentives to enhance the development of family centered, community coordinated services. But these developments bring new challenges for professionals.

The first challenge will be to train interdisciplinary professionals. Currently few programs offer curricula in assessment and intervention strategies for preschoolers. University-based preservice programs will need to expand coursework and clinical placements to fulfill the future demand for professionals. However, a greater challenge will be to upgrade the knowledge and skills of current practitioners. It will no longer be enough for special educators, nurses, physicians, occupational, physical, and speech therapists, nutritionists, and social workers to acquire competencies in their disciplines. They will now have to acquire knowledge and skills shared by professionals in other disciplines. Moreover, they will have to make joint practice decisions based on this interdisciplinary content. Many of these interdisciplinary competencies are related to preventive health and children with special health care needs.

WHY IS HEALTH CARE SO IMPORTANT TO EARLY INTERVENTION?

From a health perspective, the years between birth and 5 years of age are critical. This is the time of rapid physiological growth and development. Optimal neurological and musculo-skeletal growth is critical for the development of later cognitive, psychomotor, and speech/language skills.

The immune system, which begins with initial reliance on maternal antibodies during the first few months of life, develops antibodies which protect against the attacks of outside organisms. Listen to the parent of a toddler, and you will hear stories of frequent bouts with colds and ear infections as the baby's immune system develops resistance.

For any child, the first two years also mark the identification of many minor, or perhaps a few major, health problems. Although new parents commonly think that all conditions can be identified at the time of birth, many diseases and disabilities are not evident until well into the second year. For children with diagnosed health problems, the preschool years also represent a time when special equipment, surgeries, and therapies are needed to eliminate a medical problem, or reduce its later impact. Many of these children have no residual problems by the time they enter first grade. This situation is the ultimate goal of early intervention for all children with, or at risk for developmental disabilities.

Health care issues are increasingly important as interdisciplinary educational services become available to preschoolers and infants and toddlers with special health care needs. It is already widely recognized that group care of preschoolers is associated with increased incidence of illness in all children (Hanline & Hanson, 1989). Moreover, day care facilities have been found to present special safety hazards for children (Sells & Paeth, 1987). These risks are increased when a child is already highly susceptible to infection or injury due to a medical condition. As a result, many professionals from hospital, center-based, or home-based programs are confronting complex health care issues for the first time. Many of these health problems directly affect the child's ability to benefit from available educational and related services.

Thus, while the humanistic and developmental values of early intervention are accepted without question, it becomes imperative that interdisciplinary professionals work together to combine issues related to the health of the child and its impact on the current level of adaptive functioning. This aspect is particularly important if the child has special health care needs.

THE CHILD WITH SPECIAL HEALTH CARE NEEDS

Parents will confirm that children are special in the eyes of their parents, their siblings, and those around them. In recent years, however, the concept of special children has taken on a new meaning. Frequently, it has come to mean the child who has severe, long-term problems in adaptive functioning in cognitive, physical, psychosocial and/or self-help domains. These children often need additional help from others to function in today's society.

The term "child with special health care needs" refers to a subset of these children. These children have a physical, emotional or mental condition that interferes with their development and learning. Many times, these conditions are serious and long-term.

From an educational perspective, children with special health care needs often require special medications, treatments or appliances in order to receive optimal benefit from their school placement. For example, a child may have a tracheostomy tube for breathing, a gastrostomy tube for feeding, and a urinary catheter for passage of urine from the body. Another child may have periodic seizures, or need medication several times a day to control diabetes. Still another child may be receiving chemotherapy for cancer and receive medications through a relatively permanent tube leading directly into the heart. Regardless of the diagnosis, these children would be considered to have special health care needs.

The term "child with special health care needs" cannot be used without a word of caution. An overemphasis on "special needs" and "specialized adaptation to life" often causes professionals and parents alike to forget that even a child with special needs is a child first. The child and family have the same basic needs as other children and families. The instincts and parenting skills used with any child can be used when the child has, or is at risk for, a developmental disability or health problem. We all need to be accepted as individuals with our unique set of wishes, desires, strengths, and weaknesses. That makes us all human.

CHANGING HEALTH CARE NEEDS

Many professionals ask, "Where do children with special health care needs come from? I don't remember children like this when I was growing up." That is probably a very accurate observation, for children's health care needs have changed dramatically over the last 20 or 30 years.

Estimates on the number of children with handicapping conditions remains low compared to "normal" children; however, the incidence and prevalence of chronic illnesses in children under 18 years of age is not inconsequential. Generally, it is estimated that 10% to 15% of children under 18 years of age have some type of chronic condition, even though it may be mild. Most frequently, these conditions are respiratory, neurological (including seizures) or musculo-skeletal in nature. An estimated 1% to 1.5% have a severe chronic condition (Crowley, 1990). What is more disturbing is that incidence and prevalence rates of chronic physical conditions in children are increasing.

Several factors have contributed to these trends. First, primary prevention through vaccination and improved management of acute illnesses in children have resulted in a gradual decrease in episodic care. At the same time, improved prenatal and perinatal care and the development of sophisticated perinatal networks of primary, secondary, and tertiary health centers have meant that many infants who would have died only a few years ago are being saved. De-institutionalization has eliminated large residential groups. As a result, there are fewer concentrated epidemics, but the prevalence of chronic conditions in the general population has increased.

Medical care has also been affected by epidemics of previously unknown conditions such as pediatric AIDS and prenatal substance exposure. The federal government has allocated substantial resources to learn more about the causes and long-range consequences of these conditions.

Although the incidence and prevalence of chronic pediatric conditions has increased, so has the complexity of health needs. Children are now being discharged from hospitals on apnea monitors, ventilators, and peritoneal dialysis. Escalating hospital costs and improved technology have resulted in early discharge of even very young children who require complex care.

Commonly, these children are discharged from complex, tertiary centers into the care of their family. This means that parents must cope with the usual rigors of childrearing, as well as the additional stresses of dealing with the emotional consequences of an ill child. In addition, they must demonstrate competency in monitoring and changing ventilation equipment, recognizing subtle signs of respiratory distress, and administering cardiopulmonary resuscitation appropriately. Parents are frequently required to provide 24-hour care for their child in a home setting adapted to meet the medical needs of the ill child. This is a task many doctors and nurses would be hard-pressed to handle on a daily basis.

Philosophically, most parents prefer having the child at home with them. Indeed, generally the child does much better in the home setting. However, home care is often at great cost. Insurance companies frequently encourage home care, on the basis of greater cost effectiveness. However, their statistics do not consider extra family expenses or the consequences of lost income if one parent quits a job to stay home to care for the child. Statistics also infrequently address the strain which long hours, continuing stress, and lack of respite care can have on a family. The situation is even more complex when one realizes that many communities are unprepared to support the needs of such families. Frequently, a community does not have professionals, even physicians, who are adequately trained to meet the child's special health care needs.

IF CHILDREN HAVE SPECIAL HEALTH CARE NEEDS, WHY ARE THEY IN SCHOOL?

The difficulties families experience in meeting the special health needs of their children affects the school. Children with chronic illnesses and handicapping conditions spend more time in school than any place outside the home (Levenson & Cooper, 1984; Walker, 1984). Thus, schools are not only faced with children with greater medical complexity than ever envisioned, they are often viewed by the families as resources for technical assistance and support.

School personnel, concerned with the issues of ethics and liability consequently debate issues such as, Who has the responsibility for health care in the school setting? Who should provide this care? What professional competencies are required? What care cannot safely be provided in the school setting? What types of emergency backups are necessary? This text will address these questions.

Evolution of School-Based Services for Children with Special Health Care Needs

Historically, many children with complex health care needs were confined to institutions or lived at home, isolated in back rooms. These children seldom went to school or received private tutoring. As a result, they were not equipped to function as independent adults or to become productive members of their local communities.

As early as the 1920s, educators began to focus on the need for special education classes for children whose needs were not being met in traditional educational programs (Wang, 1989). Over the years, special education programs were developed, but integration with other children was not complete.

During that time, school health services also failed to adequately address the needs of children with medical problems. To avoid conflicts with local physicians, local health departments assumed responsibility for school health care. These departments focused on communicable disease control and absenteeism during epidemics. Since school was viewed as a place for well children, and since each child was viewed as having a medical home in the community, there was little need for extensive health care in the school environment.

From this early background, school health care evolved into the integrated components of health education, environmental management, and health services. Health education most frequently addressed basic communicable disease control, hygiene, first aid, and growth and development issues such as menstruation. This content was often not a priority. It was all too frequently relegated to a short discussion during a physical education class forced inside on a rainy day. Health education later expanded to include education for school personnel, students, and families related to specific conditions and preventive health practices.

Environmental management began with a recognition of the impact the school building and grounds could have on infection control and evolved to the present day. Guidelines were developed regarding water fountains and toilet seat construction which decreased the probability of infection spreading. Regulations were passed regarding appropriate refrigeration and cooking appliances for school kitchens, as well as laws about appropriate meal composition and food storage. Playground equipment manufacturers became more aware of safe and age-appropriate construction. Landscape architects became more sophisticated about the utilization of plants that were not harmful if touched or consumed by a child.

Health services focused primarily on accident prevention, first aid, and screening procedures to detect vision, hearing, and orthopedic problems. In a few areas, schools hired school nurses, but their role was often limited to maintaining the sick room and writing excuses to teachers for students who became ill at school.

It was assumed by all that the parent had the legal responsibility for the child. Consequently, the parent had the responsibility for all medical care. If a child was acutely ill, the parent was immediately summoned, the child was isolated, and upon parental arrival, the child was sent home. A child with a more serious illness was not allowed into the school setting. If the child was lucky, a homebound teacher/social worker made occasional home visits.

The Profound Influence of Legislation on the
Health Care of Children with Special Needs

School-based services for children with serious health problems received an invaluable boost by two pieces of landmark federal legislation, Public Law 94-142 (P.L. 94-142) and Public Law 99-457 (P.L. 99-457).

P.L. 94-142

In 1975, the Education for All Handicapped Children's Act (EHCA) was passed. That law provided for free, appropriate public education for all children from 5 to 18 years of age, even if those children had serious cognitive, physical, or psychosocial problems. A critical concept in this legislation was "placement in the least restrictive environment." For some children that environment meant placement in a regular classroom; for some, it meant mainstreaming into regular classrooms for certain activities; for some, a special education classroom; and for others, home-bound or hospital-based education. Non-discriminatory testing, Child Find (early identification of children with special needs by educational agencies), individualized educational plans, parental involvement, and due process were other critical components. The Education for All Handicapped Children's Act served as the basis for expansion of educational services to children with special needs.

Another key concept included in P.L. 94-142 was "related services." While education of the child was seen as the primary responsibility of the school, the law recognized that children with special needs would require additional services for them to maximize the benefits received from school placement. Related services, such as transportation, developmental, corrective, and supportive services were mandated in an attempt to assist a student with a handicap to benefit from special education. Specialized services such as special education, speech pathology, audiology, psychological services, and physical and occupational therapy were included. Also included were medical services for diagnosis and evaluation (Education for the Handicapped Law Report, 1984). These services were to be provided to the family at no additional cost.

Many states have experienced extensive litigation in an effort to define specific services to be included in the related services category. Issues that have been litigated include psychotherapy and counseling, transportation and recreation resources, specialized environments, and health related services (Osbourne, 1984, p. 249).

Specific litigation of health related services has shown that activities that can be performed by a school nurse or other trained person must be provided. Individual states functioning within their rights to define who is, or is not, legally permitted to perform medically related services contributed to variation in implementation of this health services mandate. As a result, courts have determined that school systems were responsible for providing clean intermittent catheterizations, health services for children with tracheostomy tubes, and similar services, if trained health personnel were permitted to perform those services under state law.

In some areas, school nurses provide these services. In other areas, the responsibility for the care of chronically ill children is shared by the school's nurse and the school's special education section (Walker, 1984). When comprehensive school health nursing services are not available, special education personnel in many states find themselves responsible for the daily management of children who are chronically ill or developmentally delayed. These services may include special feedings, suctioning, catheterizations, medications, and safety (Esterson & Bluth, 1987). As a result, teachers and other school personnel have frequently been forced to perform procedures for which they have little or no preparation or supervision.

P.L. 99-457

The Education of the Handicapped Act Amendments of 1986 (P.L. 99-457) expanded the components of P.L. 94-142 to include handicapped children from 3 to 5 years of age. Part H of that legislation provided each state with the right to choose whether to extend these services to infants and toddlers with, or at risk for, a variety of handicapping conditions. This discretionary program was allowed a four year phase-in period.

P.L. 94-142 acknowledged the concern that early physical, behavioral, and psychological problems could compromise development and learning. It further recognized that physical illness could affect early development, especially motor and social competencies, and self-help skills. Thus, health care and education were recognized as functionally inseparable (Fox, Freedman, & Klepper, 1989).

This position is supported by research documenting the effectiveness of early intervention in accelerating and maintaining developmental progress in infants who are handicapped or at risk (Bricker, Bailey, & Bruder, 1984; Castro & Mastropieri, 1986; Dunst, 1985; Dunst, Snyder, & Mankinen, 1986; Shonkoff & Hauser-Cram, 1987). Conversely, P.L. 99-457 recognized the importance of early intervention in minimizing subsequent requirements for special education and institutionalization (Public Law 99-457: Education of the Handicapped Act Amendments of 1986, Sec. 671[a]).

P.L. 99-457 also served as a catalyst in policy development. It required definitions of target populations and identified early intervention services. It also mandated policy statements regarding the goals, purposes, and outcomes of intervention activities. For the first time, the family was seen as a critical part of the child's environment, and the importance of family involvement in all aspects of the child's care was acknowledged.

The law's emphasis on family centered care and increased family involvement in all activities represented a totally new philosophy in professional/family relationships. Previously, professionals tried to diagnose what was wrong and attempt to fix it. Families were the consumers of decisions made by professionals who tried to identify what was "right for the family." The parents were "rarely the makers of decisions, no matter how intimately those decisions affected their lives" (Ziegler, 1989, p. 85).

With the advent of family centered care, professionals were required to move from the traditional prescriptive approach to a more consultative one. In this approach, the family and professional jointly identify concerns, goals, and intervention strategies. Such modifications in professional and family relationships and the acknowledgment of the important role of the family are important methods of enhancing a family's capacity to deal with the needs of their child.

In addition to providing federal funding of direct service programs, P.L. 99-457 addressed the need to establish state and local systems of care designed to provide coordinated, nonduplicative care. Interdisciplinary, interagency services were developed. Specific intervention components such as family assessment, interdisciplinary team approaches, Individualized Family Service Plans, and case management were identified as methods of providing coordinated services and individualization of care. This approach was recognized as imperative to lessen stress on the family and help family members become more independent and more integrated into their communities. Community-based, coordinated care was also viewed as more responsive to the needs of families, as well as more cost-effective and efficient.

WHAT HEALTH COMPETENCIES ARE SHARED BY ALL DISCIPLINES?

The Florida Consortium of Newborn Intervention Programs sponsored a large-scale research study of competencies necessary for eleven categories of professionals working with infants and toddlers with or at risk for developmental disabilities (Hakes, 1990). The researchers found a large number of interdisciplinary competencies related to background knowledge, identification, screening, assessment, determination of need, team processes, development of the Individualized Family Service Plan, case management, intervention and evaluation, and family supports. The demonstration of core health related knowledge was viewed to be critical for all disciplines:

1. Preconceptual risk factors;
2. Methods to prevent disease or disability (including nutrition; teen pregnancy; child abuse; maternal drug abuse; accidents; infection control; prenatal care; basic hygiene, and safety);
3. Atypical development resulting from environmental and lifestyle conditions (toxins; accidents; drug abuse; genetic abnormalities, or other perinatal risk factors);
4. Typical and atypical physical development of birth to 2-year-olds (including specific neurological disorders such as: cerebral palsy, epilepsy, and spina bifida; orthopedic problems; gross and fine skills; reflexes);
5. Medical conditions found in infants and toddlers, and their effects on development;
6. Techniques to promote physical development in typical and atypical birth to 2-year-olds;
7. Techniques to work with birth to 2-year-olds with neurodevelopmental delays & disorders;
8. Medical procedures and monitoring equipment involved in caring for a medically complex birth to 2-year-old including, but not limited to, airway management, tracheostomies, ventilator care, suctioning, and gastrostomy tubes;
9. Commonly prescribed medications;
10. Growth enhancing/inhibiting environments and strategies used to enhance growth in various settings. (Hakes, 1990).

While the competencies addressed in this study were specifically for professionals working with birth to 2-year-olds, they are equally applicable to the needs of 3- to 5-year-old children with, or at risk for, developmental disabilities.

PRACTICAL RECOMMENDATIONS FOR INTERDISCIPLINARY IMPLEMENTATION OF P.L. 99-457

The challenge of P.L. 99-457 is to put these and related competencies into practice. Currently, states are exploring ways to accomplish this goal and enhance the child's optimal development. Action plans must address not only the child's "problems and needs" but the strengths inherent in the child and family. Thus, comprehensive plans must consider developmental issues related to all children, as well as address areas of special need. While home-based or alternative placement options may be the best choice for many children, it is anticipated that most children will be optimally served in a center-based educational program. The development of such placement options requires interdisciplinary consideration of several health related areas.

The first consideration is the identification of a philosophical basis for health related programs. A key assumption is that unless optimal levels of wellness are promoted, a child's potential to function in cognitive, psychosocial, and physical development may be adversely affected (Haynes, 1983). Although children who are chronically ill or developmentally delayed may not be sick, in the common use of the term, the nature and extent of their disabilities may put them at higher risk for failure to thrive, recurrent illnesses and unwarranted secondary disabilities (Haynes, 1983, p. 5).

Second, health services should be designed to promote the child's ability to learn in the least restrictive environment, not provide primary medical care. Thus, health services should be integrated into a network of supportive services, including occupational, physical and speech therapy, audiology, special education, psychology, nutrition, and social work. These interwoven services, in concert with active parental participation, augment carefully sequenced educational plans contributing to optimal growth and development, to the extent of the individual child's abilities.

Third, health services should include direct services to children only as necessary to facilitate school attendance and individual learning, within the parameters of legislation related to state statutes for child care (for children with and without special health care needs) and legislation such as P.L. 94-142 and P.L. 99-457. This position removes the fear that schools will become health centers, rather than institutions of learning (Rustia, Hartley, Hansen, Schulte, & Spielman, 1984). Although the school may assist in maximizing health, the ultimate responsibility for the child and the child's health needs belongs to the parents.

Finally, all professionals, especially those from health and educational systems must make a concerted effort to mesh the two traditionally separate yet complementary systems into a unified approach that provides better services for children who are handicapped (Morse, 1990). General knowledge regarding chronic conditions and the management of specific health needs can facilitate this process.

BIBLIOGRAPHY

American Academy of Pediatrics. (1987). *School health: A guide for health professionals.* Elk Grove, IL: Author.

Public Law 99-457: *Education of the Handicapped Act Amendments of 1986,* Sec.671[a], 1146-1150.

2

WHAT MAKES AN INFANT OR TODDLER AT RISK?

Under the guidelines of P.L. 99-457, Part H, infants and toddlers who are handicapped are defined as children from birth to 3 years old who need early intervention services. The need for services can be based on measured delays in cognitive, physical, language, speech, psychosocial, or self-help areas. The need can also be based on classification as a child who is *at risk* for later delay.

Risk refers to an increased probability that a future event may occur. For the purposes of this text, at risk refers to a high probability that the child has or will have a delay in development. The concept of risk is based on two basic principles: (1) no disease occurs by chance; and (2) a specific disease follows a recognizable pattern. Given these two premises, a study of people with a particular condition can yield valuable information about factors shared by all of those affected. When others also have those characteristics, they are said to be at risk. That is, they are *more likely* to develop the condition or characteristics, although this does not always happen.

The identification of individuals at risk is very important from a prevention standpoint. Identification of risk factors provides opportunities for programs which lead to actual risk reduction, or early intervention opportunities for those who have already developed the risk factors.

There are generally considered to be three types of risk: established, biologic, and environmental.

ESTABLISHED RISK: DIAGNOSED CONDITION

Infants in the established risk category, (sometimes called "presumed handicapped"), have diagnosed conditions associated with later delays in development. The defect may be genetic, structural, or metabolic (von Windeguth, Urbano, Hayes, & Martyn, 1988). According to Dowds and Graham (1989), some of the most common conditions of established risk are:

1. Genetic problems (e.g., Down syndrome);
2. Neurological abnormalities or insults. (e.g., cerebral palsy);
3. Congenital and acquired diseases (e.g., infection with cytomegalovirus, and Human Immunodeficiency Virus);
4. Severe toxic exposure with manifestation in the child (e.g., Fetal Alcohol Syndrome);
5. Communication or relationship disorders (e.g., Autism, Pervasive Developmental Disability, Severe Atypical Behavior Disorder);
6. Severe vision or hearing impairments;
7. Birthweight below 1,000 grams;
8. Complex or technology dependent illnesses.

More on specific diseases is included in Chapter 3.

BIOLOGICAL RISK

Biological risk factors may be genetic in origin or relate directly to characteristics of the mother. They may also reflect events that occurred prenatally, perinatally, or postnatally. In some cases, the condition is an acquired risk which results from an event when the child is several years of age. For example, a child suffers brain trauma in a serious automobile accident at 6 years of age.

Genetic Risk Factors

This category refers to chromosomal, single gene, or multifactorial genetic problems. A family history may document diagnosed genetic problems, congenital anomalies, deafness, mental retardation, metabolic abnormalities, muscular disorders, and/or neurological disease.

Maternal Risk Factors

The characteristics of the mother have a strong influence on the environment of the developing fetus during pregnancy. There are several maternal risk factors to consider.

Age

A mother with a chronological age of less than 15 years of age is often not sufficiently physiologically developed to optimally nurture a developing baby. Consequently, teenage mothers often have premature infants or infants who die during the first two weeks of life. Maternal chronological age of over 35 years is associated with increased risk for chromosomal problems in the fetus. Down syndrome is one example.

Poverty

Americans who live in poverty are at increased statistical risk for low birthweight and infant mortality. Difficulty in receiving adequate nutrition, health care, and housing probably contribute to increased risk.

Educational Level

High educational level is closely associated with long range positive outcomes in the baby. Statistically, infants of mothers who have not completed high school or its equivalent are at increased risk for developmental delay. More educated mothers have infants with lower risks, even if the mother is very young or older, or is otherwise at statistical risk. This finding is also closely related to income level, access to health care, attitudes toward preventive health care and life style practices.

Spacing Between Pregnancies

The ideal spacing between births is about two years. When siblings are born too closely together, the mother's body does not have an adequate opportunity for recuperation.

Chronic Disease in the Mother

Diabetes, chronic high blood pressure, pulmonary disease, anemia, and heart disease can physiologically compromise the developing baby by contributing to fetal hypoxia. These maternal conditions are frequently made worse by the stress of the pregnancy.

Reproductive Problems in the Mother

Frequently, these problems are the result of uterine disease, disorders or structural problems related to the female anatomy, or the placement and/or development of the placenta. These problems can contribute to bleeding, premature delivery, or other types of fetal distress. A history of three or more spontaneous miscarriages or still-borns, infertility, or genito-urinary surgery may be related to maternal reproductive problems.

Poor Obstetrical History

Poor obstetrical history refers to complications in a previous pregnancy. It also refers to a previous delivery of an infant who was premature or ill.

Rh Incompatibility (Iso-Immunization)

Rh factor is a characteristic of human blood. Most women are Rh positive and have Rh positive children. In this situation, the mother's blood and the infant's blood are compatible and there is no problem. However, if the mother is Rh negative and the father is Rh positive, there is a chance the baby will inherit Rh positive blood. In this case, the bloods of the mother and the fetus are incompatible. The mother's body recognizes the fetal blood as a foreign substance and begins to form antibodies against it. Generally, there is insufficient maternal buildup in the first pregnancy to cause a major problem for the fetus, but incompatibility in later pregnancies may result in adverse fetal outcomes.

Non-Immune Status in the Mother

If the mother does not have adequate immunological protection, she may contract a viral infection prenatally. Many viruses, especially those contracted during the first trimester, have adverse effects on the developing fetus.

Prenatal Risk Factors

Events which occur during the pregnancy are especially important, since the majority of developmental disabilities can be linked to prenatal occurrence.

Selected Infections

Viral infections present the greatest threat to a pregnancy. The most commonly acquired viral infections fall under the acronym TORCH VIRUS (Toxoplasmosis, Other—which includes Human Immunodeficiency Virus—Rubella, Cytomegalovirus, and Hepatitis).

Substance Abuse

Maternal ingestion of a variety of substances may affect fetal development. Excessive use (abuse) increases the threat to the optimal growth and development of the fetus. Potential adverse outcomes for infants who have been exposed to drugs include low birthweight, congenital malformations, mental retardation, and seizures or strokes (Nolan, 1991). The growing problem of prenatal abuse of alcohol, cigarettes, and cocaine is of particular concern.

Prenatal Medical Conditions

Some women, with no history of chronic disease, may develop signs of diabetes, anemia, or either high or low blood pressure during a pregnancy. These signs frequently are indications of complications in the pregnancy, and should be investigated further by an obstetrician.

Inadequate Prenatal Care

Many women do not seek prenatal care until the third trimester, even when such care is easily accessible. The delay in receiving medical supervision of the pregnancy often results in increased incidence of low birthweight, and possibly avoidable complications.

Trauma

Trauma during a pregnancy may impair the body's ability to provide an optimal environment for the developing fetus or may actually lead to a miscarriage. Accidents and injuries are widely recognized sources of trauma. However, there is a growing realization that physical abuse during pregnancy has been greatly under recognized. Professionals should include screening for physical abuse as an integral part of all prenatal history and physical examinations.

Placental Problems

Structural abnormalities and abnormal functioning of the placenta contribute to the development of conditions such as placenta previa and abruptio placenta. These conditions are characterized by premature separation of the placenta from the uterine lining and frequently lead to premature delivery.

Poor Weight Gain

Twenty years ago, doctors often advised pregnant women to limit their prenatal weight gain. Today, we realize that a prenatal weight gain of 25 to 35 pounds is optimal for fetal development. Inadequate prenatal nutrition and excessive vomiting during pregnancy (hyperemesis) are frequent causes of poor weight gain.

Perinatal and Postnatal Risk Factors

While prenatal problems are the major source of later developmental delay and disability, 10% to 20% of cases of mental retardation can be traced back to problems that occur in the last two weeks of pregnancy, during labor and delivery, or are acquired during infancy or childhood.

Inadequate Oxygen (Hypoxia or Anoxia)

Conditions leading to reduced oxygen intake can result from complications during delivery (such as, an umbilical cord wrapped around the infant's neck), medical conditions contributing to low oxygen levels (such as congenital heart disease or immature infant lung development), or later accidents (such as near drowning).

Inadequate Growth

Low birthweight (less than 2,000 grams, or 5 pounds, 8 ounces at birth) and its long-term complications are widely recognized as significant risk factors. Low birthweight may occur as a result of prematurity (birth before 38 weeks gestational age) or intrauterine growth retardation. Many of these low birthweight infants suffer from neonatal problems such as intracranial hemorrhage, abnormally elevated bilirubin levels, persistent fetal circulation, neonatal seizures, and retinopathy. With intensive treatment during the neonatal period, many of these infants are able to develop normally. However, a significant number of them demonstrate cognitive delays, fine motor problems, visual perceptual difficulties, behavioral disorders, school failure, and social problems. These problems are inversely related to birthweight, with the smallest infants generally being the most involved. Major problems generally require early and ongoing intervention. Milder deficits are first identified as subtle learning disabilities or sensory processing deficits during elementary school.

Presence of Two or More Congenital Malformations

While malformations do not necessarily affect functioning, they frequently indicate underlying physiological dysfunction. Presence of such external characteristics as low-set ears indicate the need for more in-depth evaluation.

Chronic or Prolonged Illness

Long-term illness in young children may contribute to developmental delay or adversely affect current levels of adaptive functioning. Some illnesses are the result of poor anatomical development. This is the case in many types of hydrocephalus. Other illness are degenerative disorders caused by inborn metabolic errors, such as Tay Sachs and endocrine disorders. Medical regimes and hospitalizations employed to treat illness may also contribute to alterations in physiological functioning. For example, the use of mechanical ventilators in neonatal intensive care units has been associated with the development of later respiratory complications, such as Bronchopulmonary Dysplasia.

Serious Infection

Infections such as colds and childhood communicable diseases are common and generally of no long-term consequence. However, serious illnesses such as meningitis, encephalitis, generalized infection (septicemia), and pediatric AIDS are often associated with long-range neurological involvement.

Trauma

Childhood accidents are a major source of disease and disability in the United States. A growing number of incidents which, in the past, would have been classified as accidents, are now being recognized as child abuse.

ENVIRONMENTAL RISK

There is increasing realization that social, physical and behavioral factors in a child's environment can also put the child at risk by hindering optimal growth and development. Although there is no universal definition of the components of environmental risk, the following are some generally accepted factors.

Inadequate Health Care

Even when services are available, they are not always used. The lack of adequate family health care can result in inadequate primary preventive practices, failure to detect health problems early, and inadequate management of existing problems.

Inadequate Nutrition

This is associated with poor preventive health practices, and may result in or contribute to the development of health problems such as anemia. Further, inadequate nutrition in the early years of life can adversely affect optimal growth and development.

Poisons or Environmental Toxins

This includes sources of lead poisoning, cigarette smoking, toxic waste, and uncontrolled drugs and guns. These agents can adversely affect optimal growth and development directly or indirectly.

Low Socio-Economic Status

Low socio-economic status (SES) is one of the most significant variables influencing perinatal mortality and long-term morbidity. Low SES is especially notable in the presence of single parent families; teenage parents; and parents with limited financial resources, inadequate housing, and transportation.

Caregiver Who Cannot Consistently Perform Essential Parenting Functions

This factor includes caregivers with physical impairment, physical or emotional dysfunction, limited functional ability, or emotional illness, as well as those who demonstrate dysfunctional interactions, or inappropriate infant stimulation.

Presence of Physical or Emotional Abuse in the Family

Abuse is frequently more prevalent when there is a child with a handicapping condition in the family. Abuse of the child, the sibling of the child, and the spouse must all be considered.

Child is in an Institution, Foster Care or Shelter, or is a Member of a Homeless or Migrant Family

Temporary housing is often associated with other problems such as poor parental functioning, abuse or low socio-economic status. The numbers in these categories are increasing and represent evolving groups of children at increased risk.

INTERACTION OF VARIABLES

It should be noted that the presence of risk factors does not automatically mean the child will have problems. However, risk factors do mean an increased probability. When several variables exist at the same time, they frequently interact and greatly increase the risk of either alone. For this reason, interdisciplinary professionals need to expand traditional emphasis on established conditions and biological risks to include the influence of psychosocial factors.

3

WHAT MEDICAL PROBLEMS AM I MOST LIKELY TO ENCOUNTER?

O ne of the greatest challenges of caring for children with special health needs is simply learning more about their medical conditions. This chapter will provide a description of some of the most common conditions, the cause of each, and common health problems associated with that condition. The reader is cautioned to consider each child as an individual. Focus on each child's current level of adaptive functioning rather than only on the diagnosis.

CEREBRAL PALSY

Description

Cerebral palsy is a term used to describe symptoms associated with different conditions rather than one specific disease. It describes a group of symptoms including paralysis, muscle weakness, and lack of coordination of the motor system.

There are several types of cerebral palsy. Spastic cerebral palsy is the most common. It is characterized by stiffness or high muscle tone (hypertonicity); poor control over posture, balance, and muscle coordination; and a persistence of primitive reflexes. These persistent primitive reflexes make it difficult forthe child to control involuntary muscle movement and progress to coordinated motor tasks such as eating, swallowing, sitting, and walking. A child with this type of cerebral palsy will show increased or decreased resistance to passive movement. The child may arch the back in an exaggerated fashion. The spasticity in the lower extremities may make diapering difficult.

The second type of cerebral palsy is athetoid (dyskinetic cerebral palsy). This type is characterized by abnormal involuntary, uncontrolled movements. Typically, these are slow, wormlike, writhing movements that involve the entire body, including the neck, facial muscles, and tongue. Choreoathetosis describes jerky, abrupt movements. Dystonia describes slow, rhythmic movements of the entire body or extremity. These involuntary movements are increased when the child is anxious or is attempting voluntary movement.

Ataxia cerebral palsy is the least common type. It is characterized by irregular muscle action and poor muscle coordination. Disturbed sense of balance and depth perception are usually present. As a result, the child may develop a broad-based, lurching gait and experience difficulty standing and walking.

Many children have a mixed type of cerebral palsy. This is most commonly a combination of spasticity and athetosis. These children have a great deal of neurological involvement.

Cause

Cerebral palsy is caused by injury to the brain. This injury can occur during fetal growth, labor and delivery, or infancy and childhood. The most common cause of injury is inadequate oxygen. Damage from intracranial hemorrhage or perinatal infection, prematurity, brain malformation, endocrine abnormalities, and teratogenic exposure are implicated as causes. Cerebral palsy may also occur as the result of a head injury or child abuse. Often, no exact cause can be identified for a particular child.

Children with cerebral palsy have normal muscles and nerves. Their neuro-muscular problems develop as a result of brain damage and subsequent loss of the brain's ability to control muscle action. The extent of the cerebral palsy is dependent on the type of brain injury, when it occurred, and the exact location of brain involvement. The resultant muscle involvement may be mild or severe. Although the brain damage is not progressive, cerebral palsy cannot be cured. However, early intervention and therapy may help alleviate the symptoms.

Diagnosis

The diagnosis of cerebral palsy is largely based on clinical findings. Sometimes laboratory tests are done to provide supporting evidence of low oxygen levels or specific brain damage due to hemorrhage. However, these tests are confirmatory rather than diagnostic.

Because the diagnosis is based on clinical findings, it is often delayed until the child is 12 to 18 months old. At this time, a diagnosis can be based on the child's failure to achieve normal developmental milestones as well as observation of abnormal movement patterns. Delayed motor milestones are particularly significant if other milestones such as language and personal-social development are normal.

Common Health Problems

Related health problems are also dependent on the part of the brain that has been damaged and the extent of involvement. Children with cerebral palsy are at risk for many of the following health problems.

Seizures

Seizure activity may be very complex and difficult to control due to severe brain damage. Most frequently, seizure activity involves generalized tonic-clonic seizures (grand mal). For further discussion of seizures, refer to the earlier section in this chapter and the section on seizure management in Chapter 6.

Feeding Difficulties

Since the motor disorders inherent in cerebral palsy affect the muscles in the tongue, lips, jaws, and upper esophagus, feeding problems are common. The child should be evaluated by a team of feeding specialists to assess skills related to biting, chewing, and swallowing.

Poor Nutrition and Growth

Difficulties in feeding and excessive caloric demands as a result of constant motor movement occur frequently in cerebral palsy. Therefore, inadequate nutrition and poor growth may result.

Musculo-Skeletal Complications

The presence of involuntary movements means that children with cerebral palsy may need assistance from others, or special equipment to gain greater independence in motor activities, dressing, and feeding.

This special equipment helps to promote more normalized postures and reduce complications.

At times, the predominance of certain muscle groups contributes to the development of abnormal musculo-skeletal conditions such as hip dislocations, tight heel cords, or contractures. Scoliosis and limps may also occur as a result of muscle imbalance. Many of these complications require orthopedic evaluation and/or later surgery.

Bowel Problems

Poor muscle tone, inactivity, and feeding difficulties can contribute to the development of constipation, encopresis, and bowel dysfunction. Sufficient levels of dietary roughage, fluids, and regular bowel training are often helpful.

Visual Problems

Muscle imbalance also affects the eyes. As a result, many children with cerebral palsy suffer from strabismus (malalignment of the eyes resulting in visual disturbance). Special eye exercises and/or surgery may be prescribed. Other vision problems are also common, and prescriptive glasses may be necessary.

Impairment of Speech

Lack of muscle control leads to slow, labored, difficult speech. Special adaptive devices, such as lap boards, can often facilitate communication.

Hearing Problems

Certain types of brain damage, such as brain infection and excessive levels of bilirubin, can contribute to hearing problems. Many children with cerebral palsy are also susceptible to frequent infections, including middle ear infections. Hearing should be evaluated periodically to determine degree of acuity.

Learning Difficulties

For many children with cerebral palsy, learning is difficult. Motor skills, positioning, balance, and energy expenditure become real obstacles. Often their normal intelligence is hidden by their severe muscle involvement. Unfortunately, many other children have also sustained brain damage that has lead to some degree of cognitive delay.

Behavioral Problems

Infants with cerebral palsy often demonstrate exaggerated startle responses, making them over-reactive to mild stimulation. This behavior can make routine child care very difficult.

Older children can experience high levels of frustration and fatigue as a result of difficulties in motor control, perception, and communication. As a result, children with cerebral palsy often become irritable, frustrated, and seemingly uncooperative. Patience and assistive devices help reduce frustration levels.

Manifestations of attention deficit disorder may accompany cerebral palsy. Symptoms include poor attention span, hyperactivity, and distractibility (Whaley & Wong, 1987).

Infections

Since the respiratory muscles are less efficient, children with cerebral palsy are prone to upper respiratory infections. At times, these infections can be related to aspiration of fluids or food during feeding. Respiratory status and signs of possible infections should be carefully monitored. Contact the parents and physician if signs of infection are noted.

Additional Resources

To learn more about cerebral palsy, you may wish to contact the organizations listed in the Appendix.

COCAINE-EXPOSED INFANTS

Description

The use of cocaine in the United States has increased dramatically in recent years. An increasing number of women use cocaine during pregnancy and deliver infants who have been prenatally exposed to cocaine.

The association between prenatal cocaine exposure and the incidence of congenital anomalies has been inconclusive (von Windeguth & Urbano, 1989). A more serious problem seems to be the influence of cocaine on later learning and behavior.

Cocaine-exposed infants do not suffer the neonatal withdrawal and intrauterine growth retardation found in infants of opiate abusers (Chasnoff, Bussey, Savich & Stack, 1986). However, they do demonstrate tremulousness and increased startle responses (Chasnoff, Bussey, Savich, & Stack, 1986). Neurological abnormalities such as irritability and muscular rigidity have been noted (LeBlanc, Parekh, Naso, & Glass, 1987). These infants may have jerky or stiff movements, tremors in the extremities, and/or increased muscle tone.

Cause

Cocaine taken by the mother during the prenatal period easily passes from the maternal placenta to the fetus. It is metabolized into norcocaine and is believed to continue to circulate in the fetal system, rather than being returned to the mother's system for ultimate excretion.

Norcocaine acts as a central nervous system stimulant. This central nervous system stimulation results in changes in the fetal heart rate, circulatory system, and blood pressure. The exact physiological effects are now being researched.

Health Problems

Although maternal cocaine's adverse effects on the fetus are documented, the long-range impact of cocaine exposure is not clear (Kelley, Walsh, & Thompson, 1991). However, there is great concern that difficulties in organization of behavior may adversely influence later learning. Organizational difficulties are reflected in both irritability and relational problems.

Cocaine-exposed infants demonstrate disturbed sleeping patterns, and are frequently difficult to arouse. When awake, they are very irritable. This irritability extends to activities of daily living. Many cocaine-exposed infants have poor feeding patterns. They are frequently orally defensive and show aversion to someone touching them near the mouth. Basic daily feeding routines become long and laborious. Feeding becomes a time of frustration for both infant and caregiver.

Infants who have been exposed to cocaine are difficult to console. The high degree of irritability limits the infant's ability to learn from auditory or visual stimuli. This is believed to be the basis for the development of later language and articulation problems. In turn, delayed communication skills hinder later learning.

Irritability also influences the degree to which an infant or child can focus attention on a task. Many caregivers describe cocaine-exposed children as being much more hyperactive than the traditional hyperactive child. Tremors and extraneous movement further hinder the development of fine muscle skills and visual motor skills.

Difficulty in maintaining organizational states influences care-giving. The baby may give poor cues to caregivers regarding basic needs, and may be unresponsive to caring behaviors of the parents. These responses adversely affect the development of optimal recipro-cal relationships between the infant and the caregiver.

Older children demonstrate difficulty in behavioral state regulation through difficulty controlling behavior, which may change quickly from apathy to aggression. These rapid behavioral changes can lead to frustration on the part of the caregiver, and put the child at risk for child abuse or neglect.

Relational problems can be seen in older children who are unable to respond to positive reinforcement from adults in school settings. These children may also have difficulty working or playing with stu-dents or with teachers.

It is unclear how long difficulties with motor and behavioral control persist. Follow-up studies of cocaine-exposed infants have found that many motor problems persisted to four months of age. The difficulties lessened with age, but had not totally disappeared by eight months of age (Schneider, Griffith, & Chasnoff, 1989). Longitudinal research studies are currently being conducted to learn more about the long-term outcomes of cocaine exposure.

For the present, childcare workers must be sensitive to the existence of the problem in all socio-economic groups. Careful assessments must be conducted when an infant is noted to be highly irritable or difficult to console, to rule out the presence of neuro-motor problems. Prompt identification and early intervention may prevent the development of secondary problems. Care must also be taken to provide quiet, soothing environments and to use techniques designed to comfort irritable infants and children.

Additional Resources

To learn more about cocaine-exposed infants, you may wish to contact the organizations listed in the Appendix.

DOWN SYNDROME

Description

Down syndrome is a collection of symptoms (a syndrome) com-monly found in individuals who share a specific chromosomal abnormality (most commonly Trisomy 21). Down syndrome is associated with mental retardation and a set of characteristic physical attributes. While these physical characteristics may vary slightly, they generally include: small, round head with a flattened back of the head; small stature; poor muscle tone; hyperflexibility of joints; upward slant to the eyes, epicanthal folds in the inner eye corners; low-set ears; small nose and mouth; often seen with the mouth ajar and a protruding tongue; short neck; short, broad hands with a single palmar crease (and often an incurving fifth finger); and a gap between the first and second toes. Genitalia may be small and testes undescended. While initial symptoms may be very subtle, children with Down syndrome show slower motor and intellectual development as they grow. While ultimate intellectual development varies, most children are generally found to test in the mild to moderately retarded range.

Cause

Down syndrome occurs in approximately 1 in 600 live births, making it one of the most commonly occurring genetic syndromes. Down syndrome results from one of several types of chromosomal problems.

Normally, there are 2 chromosomes for each of the 22 autosomes. The majority of the time, Down syndrome results from an extra Chromosome 21 (i.e., Trisomy 21). This type of Down syndrome occurs equally in all races and socio-economic groups and is not inherited.

Trisomy 21 is the result of an error in cell division, although it is not clearly understood why this error occurs. It has been widely observed that the occurrence of Trisomy 21 is related to increased maternal age. The probability of occurrence increases significantly when a mother reaches 35 years of age and accelerates dramatically after that age. Thus, some theorists have associated syndrome incidence with aging maternal eggs. However, almost one third of all chromosomal problems can be linked to the father.

Due to the high probability of occurrence of Trisomy 21 in older mothers, prenatal genetic testing is recommended. This testing can be accomplished in two ways. Maternal alpha-fetoprotein screening involves a maternal blood test during the 12th to 14th week of pregnancy to detect abnormal levels of alpha-fetoprotein. Alpha-fetoprotein is a compound produced by the fetus. It diffuses from the fetus into the amniotic fluid and ultimately into the mother's blood supply. This is an effective screening test but is not as reliable as amniocentesis. Amniocentesis involves insertion of a needle into the fetal sac during the 14th to 16th weeks of pregnancy. The needle is used to withdraw a specimen to test alpha-fetoprotein levels as well as to study the actual chromosomes.

Some types of Down syndrome are not caused by Trisomy 21. One of these variations is a hereditary chromosomal translocation. Such translocations result from a piece of the pair of Chromosome 21 breaking off and becoming attached to another chromosome. A second variation is mosaicism. This term indicates that some of the cells of the body have an extra chromosome 21, but not all cells are affected. The percentage of affected cells in the body determines the degree to which symptoms of Down syndrome are apparent.

Some types of Down syndrome are inherited and some are not. Therefore, it is imperative that the diagnosis be based on chromosomal analysis by a genetic laboratory rather than on physical findings alone. If an inheritable type of Down syndrome is determined, the parents should be referred to a genetic counseling department, usually found at a tertiary medical center.

Common Health Problems

Heart Defects and Disease

About one-third of all children with Down syndrome suffer from a congenital heart defect. Some of these problems may resolve themselves or may result in only a heart murmur which is monitored by the physician. Other defects may be more serious and require corrective surgery.

In early life, cardiac problems may adversely affect the child's ability to get adequate oxygen. As a result, the child may tire very easily or be a poor feeder. The child may not tolerate temperature changes. Paleness in the fingernails or around the mouth may also be indications that the child is not getting enough oxygen. This is not a medical emergency, but the child should be referred to a nurse or physician for further evaluation.

Prevention of infection of the heart (subacute bacterial endocarditis) is an important consideration when a child has a heart problem. Many doctors recommend that preventive antibiotics be given prior to any dental, surgical, or invasive procedure to prevent cardiac infection.

Gastrointestinal Tract Abnormalities

Many children with Down syndrome have congenital abnormalities of the digestive tract. These structural problems may result in recurrent vomiting or symptoms of intestinal obstruction. This condition is very painful and requires immediate medical evaluation.

Chronic constipation is also a frequent problem. This is aggravated by poor muscle tone and limited exercise. Adequate roughage and fluid intake combined with exercise help control the tendency toward constipation. Due to the possibility of structural abnormalities, more severe constipation problems should be referred to the physician for comprehensive evaluation.

Frequent Infections

Most children with Down syndrome possess a compromised immune response. As a result, they are at increased risk for infection. Most commonly, children have frequent, repeated, and chronic pneumonia, tonsillitis, and ear infections. These infections are often complicated by pulmonary hypertension, frequent upper airway obstruction, and decreased alveoli (Cooney & Thurlbeck, 1982; Rowland, Nordstrom, Bean, & Burkhardt, 1981).

Children with Down syndrome also suffer from frequent skin infections. The severely dry skin experienced by some children with Down syndrome may contribute to these infections. Moisturizing products may help. If they do not, the child should be referred to the physician to rule out dry skin due to thyroid dysfunction.

The higher susceptibility to infections and difficulty in fighting off infections contribute to increased death rates. Compromised immune systems are also believed to place children with Down syndrome at higher risk for developing leukemia and autoimmune problems such as thyroid dysfunction.

Any child in a preschool setting is at increased risk for infection. The diagnosis of Down syndrome should alert professionals that a child is at an even greater risk. Aggressive preventive measures are necessary. Proper technique in handwashing and diaper changing is imperative.

Increased susceptibility means that routine colds should not be ignored. Professionals must be particularly alert for signs of infection, high temperature, listlessness, or increased breathing and pulse rates. Such symptoms indicate the need for further medical evaluation.

Antibiotics are frequently prescribed to treat infections. It is critical that antibiotics be given in the right dose and with the prescribed time intervals. This regime may necessitate that professionals give medication to the child during the school day. Remember, incompletely treated infections may be even more dangerous than untreated ones. Symptoms are often masked, but permanent damage may occur.

It should be noted that children with Down syndrome are hospitalized frequently for serious infections or surgeries. Upon returning to the school setting, the child may demonstrate a regression in previously acquired developmental skills or may tire more easily. Frequently, medications or treatments have been changed during the hospitalization. Be sure to contact the physician regarding any changes prior to the child's readmission to school. Allow the child plenty of time to fully recuperate before a full program is reinstituted.

Thyroid Problems

Low thyroid problems are frequently found in individuals with Down syndrome. Their occurrence increases with age. Since the clinical symptoms of low thyroid are similar to those of Down syndrome, thyroid studies are generally recommended for infants with Down syndrome to assure detection of thyroid dysfunction.

Genital / Urinary Abnormalities

Many males with Down syndrome have a small penis and below normal testicular volume. This is thought to be progressive from infancy to adolescence and be related to later male sterility. In addition, many males have abnormal positioning of the urinary meatus (external opening). Related internal organs are generally found to be normal.

Eye Problems

The apparent abnormalities in the development of the face contribute to a variety of eye problems. Crossing of the eyes, nearsightedness, and farsightedness are well documented. Abnormal eye movements and jerkiness are also common. Baseline and routine vision screenings are very important parts of early detection and subsequent intervention.

Ear Problems

Improper development of the face also contributes to structural abnormalities of the nose and ears. Speech problems are frequently reported. Small ear canals are frequently noted and contribute to the development of excessive accumulations of wax in the ear canal. Hearing deficits and frequent infections are common. Antibiotics and surgical interventions such as myringotomies and tubes are often prescribed to reduce the incidence of ear infections.

Structural Abnormalities Affecting Speech and Feeding

Hearing problems and abnormal development of the head contribute to delays in speech development. Physical anomalies such as underdevelopment of the maxilla and abnormal tongue size, in concert with facial and oral hypotonia, contribute to poor feeding abilities. Aggressive feeding programs are responsible for a high probability for future independent eating skills.

An increasing number of plastic surgeons are attempting "normalization" of facial characteristics such as large tongue, open mouth, and epicanthal folds. Such surgeries lead to greater social acceptance. They also contribute to improvements in nose breathing and speech, and decreased drooling.

Neuro-Muscular Problems

Children with Down syndrome follow the normal content and sequence of gross motor development, only they do it more slowly. Ultimate attainment is dependent on the degree of hypotonia (poor muscle tone) and hyperreflexia (increased extensibility of the joints). Hypotonia and hyperreflexia frequently result in problems of maintaining appropriate posture and gait. Early and aggressive physical therapy has been shown to be very effective.

Musculo-Skeletal Problems

Muscle hypotonia and hyperreflexia also contribute to the development of orthopedic problems. One of the most significant is known as atlantoaxial subluxation. This is an instability of the space between the first two cervical vertebrae which may contribute to spinal cord injury in a small percentage of children. Many physicians recommend a routine cervical spine x-ray by the time the child is 2 years old and a medical evaluation of any symptoms of neck discomfort or spasticity. Children with Down syndrome should also be evaluated for possible vertebral problems prior to exercises such as tumbling which may result in neck injury. It should be noted that most children show no evidence of such problems and can participate in all physical education activities safely.

Other musculo-skeletal problems such as scoliosis and instability of the lower lumbar vertebrae have been observed. Probably one of the most commonly reported musculo-skeletal problems in children with Down syndrome is flat feet.

Obesity

A tendency toward obesity is commonly noted in children with Down syndrome. Reduced exercise tolerance due to neuro-muscular or cardiac problems often combines with a tendency toward obesity.

The presence of hypothyroidism further contributes to excessive weight gain. As a result, major difficulties with weight control develop with both medical and social consequences. Comprehensive nutritional evaluation and monitoring of intake and weight are essential. Team discussions should also be conducted to develop individual plans for exercise programs to supplement other weight control measures.

Additional Resources

To learn more about Down syndrome, you may wish to contact the organizations listed in the Appendix.

HYDROCEPHALUS

Description

Hydrocephalus is a term that comes from the words "hydro" which means water, and "cephalus" which refers to the brain. It refers to a condition in which there is an abnormal accumulation of cerebrospinal fluid in the brain.

Cerebrospinal fluid is a clear, watery liquid that is produced in a part of the brain called the ventricles. The fluid is replaced every 6 hours, and circulates throughout the brain and spinal cord, and then is reabsorbed. Cerebrospinal fluid offers protection to the system by serving as a buffer against sudden pressure changes. It also serves as a source of nutrition and waste removal.

In normal circulation, the fluid is produced in a part of the brain called the ventricles. These ventricles are located deep in the brain and are shaped like a thumb and forefinger. (See Figure 3-1 for a picture of the ventricles.) Normally, the cerebrospinal fluid drains into the third ventricle and then into the fourth ventricle. A small amount of fluid coats the surface of the brain. However, most of the fluid drains from the fourth ventricle into the meninges which surrounds the spinal cord and is reabsorbed at the base of the spine and around the surface of the brain.

When something interferes with the normal production and flow of cerebrospinal fluid, there is an increased accumulation within the ventricles of the brain. If hydrocephalus is untreated, there is a gradual accumulation of fluid in the brain. This leads to excessive pressure inside the head, frequently increased head size (enlarged head circumference), and ultimately, brain damage.

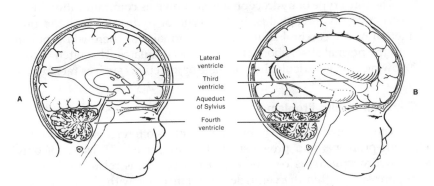

A: Patent Cerebrospinal Fluid Circulation
B: Enlarged Lateral and Third Ventricles Caused By Obstruction of Circulation-Stenosis of Aquaduct of Sylvius

Figure 3-1. Hydrocephalus: A block in the flow of cerebrospinal fluid. Reproduced with permission from Whaley, Lucille F., and Wong, Donna L.: *Nursing care of infants and children*, ed. 4, St. Louis, 1991; Mosby-Year Book, Inc.

Cause

Hydrocephalus can be associated with several medical diagnoses. It is perhaps most commonly associated with spina bifida, since the majority of infants with that diagnosis develop hydrocephalus within the first year of life.

Hydrocephalus is categorized by cause. The first type is hydrocephalus caused by an actual overproduction of cerebral spinal fluid. This overproduction is often due to a problem with the choroid plexus (the part of the brain where the cerebrospinal fluid is made). The second cause of hydrocephalus is known as noncommunicating or obstructive hydrocephalus. In this type of hydrocephalus, the actual amount of cerebral spinal fluid that is produced may be normal, but there is an obstruction in the pathways through which the cerebral spinal fluid flows. As a result, there is an accumulation of the cerebral spinal fluid within the brain's ventricles. Frequently, this type of obstruction results from a tumor or malformation such as aqueductal stenosis or Arnold Chiari malformation. In an Arnold Chiari malformation, part of the brain is compressed into the foramen magnum (an opening at the base of the skull through which the spinal cord usually passes). Since the internal connections of the brain are intact, intelligence is normal. If the displacement of the brain is severe, the child may develop respiratory distress or may need surgery.

The third type of hydrocephalus is known as communicating (non-obstructive) hydrocephalus. In this type of hydrocephalus, the production of the cerebral spinal fluid is normal, but there is a problem with the normal absorption. Thus, fluid accumulates. This often occurs following intraventricular hemorrhage or infections such as meningitis.

Common Health Problems

The underlying cause of hydrocephalus is often responsible for the health problems and prognosis a child may have. However, if only the hydrocephalus is considered, health problems relate to developing pressure within the ventricles and difficulties with shunt function.

Signs of Hydrocephalus in a Child Under 2 Years of Age

In an infant, signs of hydrocephalus may not initially result in significant intracranial pressure. This is because the child's skull bones are not fully fused. Excessive pressure in the brain is prevented because the brain can expand against the cranial bones. Thus, increasing head size, as measured by sequential measurements of head circumference, is often an early sign of hydrocephalus. Related signs may include the following: a large forehead; enlarged scalp veins; a bulging fontanel (soft spot in the top of a baby's head); irritability and sluggishness. If the condition is untreated, increasing intracranial pressure may contribute to a characteristic condition known as "Sunset Gaze" in which the eyes have a downward gaze, with the whites of the eyes being more visible than normal. Increasing intracranial pressure may also lead to vomiting, increased muscle tone, possible seizures, and coma.

Signs of Hydrocephalus in a Child Over 2 Years of Age

In children over 2 years of age, increasing head circumference is not the first sign of hydrocephalus. Since the skull bones have already fused by this age, the increasing intracranial pressure may go undetected. Thus, it is important for professionals to constantly look for the following signs: lethargy; nausea and vomiting; severe headaches; decreased level of activity; nystagmus (constant, involuntary movement of the eyeball), and seizures. Although these conditions may be associated with many conditions of varying severity, they should be noted and the cause determined.

Diagnosis

The diagnosis of hydrocephalus is often a clinical one. In young children, diagnosis is based on increasing head circumference over time and a bulging fontanel. Ultrasound can be used if the child is old enough for skull bones to have fused. More sophisticated testing procedures such as Computerized Axial Tomography (CAT Scan) and Magnetic Resonance Imaging (MRI) can be diagnostic, but are expensive and not always used in making a diagnosis.

Treatment

Treatment of hydrocephalus is focused on correcting the cause, if it can be determined. Surgical correction of an obstruction and the use of drugs or surgery to reduce the production of cerebrospinal fluid are commonly used treatment approaches.

Perhaps the most widely used treatment for hydrocephalus is the use of a shunt. Shunts are plastic tubes with a one way valve. They are surgically implanted under the child's skin. There is no external contact with the valve or the tubing. Sometimes the shunt tubing may be seen under the skin behind the ear or under the skin of the neck. After healing is completed, the shunt does not require special dressings or daily care. The child is able to engage in normal activities, although sports with potential of direct head injury may be discouraged.

There are two types of shunts (see Figure 3-2). The first is called a Ventriculoatrial Shunt (or AV shunt). One end of the shunt is placed in the ventricle of the brain where the cerebrospinal fluid is accumulating. The other is placed in the right atrium of the heart. Extra fluid is drawn off via the shunt and "shunted" to the heart, where it is absorbed via the bloodstream.

The second type of shunt is the Ventriculoperitoneal Shunt (VP Shunt). In this shunt, one end of the tube is placed in the ventricle of the brain, and the other is placed in the abdominal or peritoneal cavity. Shunted cerebrospinal fluid is reabsorbed by the lining of the cavity. Because there is more space in the peritoneal cavity than in the heart, there is room for the doctor to place longer than necessary tubing. The excess tubing is coiled up in the cavity for storage. As the child grows, the extra tubing is stretched out as necessary. This technique is advantageous because repeated surgeries to insert longer pieces of tubing can be avoided.

A small percentage of children outgrow their need for a shunt in the first years of life. However, most children require a shunt for the rest of their lives. With a properly functioning shunt, a child's prognosis is very good, but recognition of signs of complications is essential.

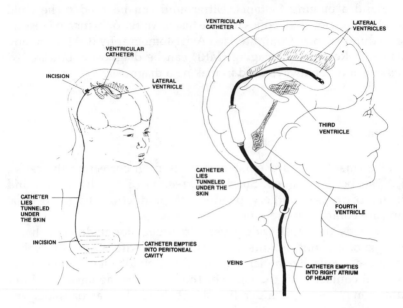

A: Ventriculo-Peritoneal Shunt   B: Ventriculo-Atrial Shunt

Figure 3-2. Shunts. From: *Shunts.* 1989. Association for Brain Tumor Research, Chicago. Reproduced with permission.

Short-Term Health Problems

Short-term health problems relate to infection of the shunt and increasing buildup of fluid in the ventricles as a result of infection or blockage. Refer to Chapter 6 for a detailed discussion of monitoring a shunt and early identification of complications.

Long-Term Health Problems

Long-term health problems are highly dependent on the severity of the underlying diagnosis. If one considers long-term prognosis, regardless of specific underlying diagnosis, several trends can be noted.

1. About 20% of infants outgrow their need for shunts during the first year (Epstein, 1984). Other children may need a shunt for life.
2. If the hydrocephalus is uncomplicated and treated early, the children have a good prognosis.
3. Some children experience normal or borderline intelligence, usually due to difficulty in reasoning. Final cognitive ability is associated with the cause of the hydrocephalus.

4. Some children have vision problems (gaze and movement) that also affect school performance.
5. If the child has a Ventriculoatrial Shunt, antibiotics should be given prior to, the day of, and after dental work and invasive procedures, to prevent infection.
6. Seizures may be associated with hydrocephalus, especially if it was due to brain tumors or infection.

Additional Resources

To learn more about hydrocephalus, you may wish to contact the organizations listed in the Appendix.

PEDIATRIC AIDS

Description

AIDS stands for Acquired Immunodeficiency Syndrome. Pediatric AIDS is the most severe pediatric manifestation of symptoms ranging from a viral infection through general, subtle symptoms (formerly called AIDS Related Complex or ARC) to a formalized definition of pediatric AIDS.

Cause

AIDS is caused by infection by the Human Immunodeficiency Virus (HIV). Pediatric AIDS refers to infection in children (under 13 years of age). The incidence is roughly evenly divided between boys and girls. Black and Hispanic children are statistically over represented among ethnic groups.

The majority of children contract HIV infection as a result of prenatal or perinatal exposure from an infected mother. A smaller percentage of children contract HIV infection through contaminated blood exposure during a transfusion or contact with infected blood products. These methods of transmission are contrasted with HIV infection in adults which is spread through exposure to infected semen, vaginal fluids, and blood.

The HIV virus is not easily transmitted. There has been no proven spread by insects; casual contacts in schools, preschools or daycare centers or workplaces; blood donation; contact with saliva, sweat or tears; eating in restaurants; swimming in public pools; or by shaking hands, sneezing or coughing. The virus is also not easily spread during caregiving activities such as diapering or feeding, or even providing direct care for a child with HIV infection.

Common Health Problems

The health problems experienced by HIV-infected infants and children are, in part, dependent on the stage of the illness.

Asymptomatic Phase

This is the period of time from actual exposure to the virus to blood changes in the child. During this period, there are generally few or no symptoms.

Whereas it may take up to 10 years for an adult to develop antibodies against the HIV virus, changes can be detected in children from 6 weeks to 1 year after exposure. When exposed to the HIV virus during the mother's pregnancy, a newborn baby may appear normal. It may be difficult to test an infant for HIV exposure, because the baby may carry maternal antibodies for months. This situation makes it difficult to determine if the child is also infected and whether the mother was the only affected person.

Early Symptoms

An HIV-infected baby may start showing symptoms within a few weeks or months, with most showing symptoms by 24 months of age. The earlier the symptoms appear, the more involved the child's symptoms will become.

Symptoms of HIV infection and AIDS in children are very different than those seen in adults. Initial symptoms may be very subtle. They may include the following: fever; failure to thrive; weight loss; enlarged liver; enlarged spleen and/or lymph nodes. These symptoms are also seen in a variety of other conditions. Consequently, their presence should indicate the need for further diagnostic testing to rule out HIV-positive status.

Pediatric AIDS

As the disease progresses, symptoms become more severe. Many children have frequent infections including persistent thrush and diarrhea. A large number of children have an unusual type of lung problem called lymphoid interstitial pneumonitis. These children also have frequent secondary infections such as Pneumocystis carinii pneumonia, cytomegalovirus, bacterial urinary tract infections, and fungus infections.

As the infection progresses, affected children show lack of attainment of developmental milestones or even regress in developmental skills. These developmental delays are often the result of progressive neurological disease. Subsequent findings often include progressive symmetrical motor deficits. Impaired brain growth affects intellectual abilities. Later symptoms include the development of secondary cancers and severe multisystem problems, often involving the liver, heart, kidney, and blood.

The diagnosis of pediatric AIDS is very specific and based on specialized laboratory tests and clinical symptoms. Currently, new laboratory tests are being developed in the hopes that affected children can be identified earlier.

Management of Symptoms

Management activities are very individualized. Not all children have all symptoms. Experimental use of antiviral agents at earlier stages of the disease appears to somewhat slow the development and severity of the symptoms. Ultimately, it is hoped that more severe symptoms can be moderated.

General management strategies include prevention of infection spread, aggressive treatment of infection with antibiotics and antipyretics (fever lowering medications), well balanced nutritional and fluid intake, good skin care to prevent skin breakdown into sores, and practicing of Universal Precautions to prevent the spread of infection to others. (See Chapter 8 for further discussion of Universal Precautions.) Children with HIV infection and AIDS are particularly sensitive to certain viruses such as chickenpox, so contact with children with chickenpox should be avoided. Children with HIV infection and pediatric AIDS should receive a modified schedule of immunizations to protect them from other childhood illnesses (see chapter 7).

Children with HIV infection and pediatric AIDS are in great need of family and community support. Needs for support are broadly based: confidentiality; nondiscrimination; housing; health education; financial assistance; family counseling; child care; transportation; respite and care coordination. Many families are functioning at the poverty level, with all of its socio-economic consequences. In addition, there is frequently an affected mother in the home, who may be too sick herself to care properly for the child. Close collaboration between school personnel and community resources can do much to assist the family in dealing with these serious obstacles.

Additional Resources

To learn more about pediatric AIDS, you may wish to contact the organizations listed in the Appendix.

MUSCULAR DYSTROPHY

Description

Muscular dystrophy (MD) is the largest single group of childhood progressive muscle diseases. Children with most types of muscular dystrophy appear to be normal at birth. Severe types like Duchenne muscular dystrophy are apparent in preschool years. Other types are not noticeable until adulthood.

Muscle weakness begins in the extremities, and additional muscles groups are affected as the disease progresses. Often, a problem is first suspected when a child has difficulty with large muscle activities such as climbing stairs or getting up from a lying position. Even a child who is initially ambulatory will probably lose the ability to ambulate by late childhood or early adolescence. There is no effective treatment for muscular dystrophy. For most types of muscular dystrophy, death occurs by early adulthood.

Cause

Muscular dystrophies are genetic in origin. Some, like Duchenne muscular dystrophy, are inherited in an X-linked pattern. Thus, only males are affected. Others may be either autosomal dominant or recessive. These types affect both sexes.

Muscular dystrophies share progressive loss of muscle function. They vary in the muscles that are affected, how the disease progresses, and when it first becomes noticeable. Diagnosis is based on decreased reflexes, elevated muscle enzymes (indicating muscle damage), and abnormal muscle function. The diagnosis is confirmed by muscle biopsy.

Health Problems

Muscle Weakness

Muscle weakness, fatigue, swelling (pseudo-hypertrophy), and cramps are major symptoms. The muscle weakness starts in the large muscle groups of the extremities. Children have difficulty holding their hands up against gravity and walking or standing. A characteristic waddling gait develops. Ultimately, the chest muscles, and the respiratory and cardiac muscles are affected. The child usually dies of respiratory or cardiac failure.

Skeletal Deformities

Contracture deformities of hip, knees, and ankles often result from increasing muscle weakness. Orthopedic evaluation is indicated for management of these secondary conditions.

Respiratory Infections

Since respiratory muscles are less effective, air exchange becomes gradually poorer. The number of respiratory infections increase. As the respiratory muscles become more involved, even mild respiratory illnesses may become very serious. Prompt medical evaluation is indicated.

Obesity

As muscles deteriorate, they are replaced with adipose tissue. In addition, loss of ambulation resulting from restricted physical activity leads to weight gain. Obesity frequently results.

Cardiac Problems

As the muscles of the heart are involved, the heart becomes less efficient. Cardiac overload and failure results.

Bowel Problems

Muscle weakness can result in poor bowel motility and constipation. Increased fluid intake, dietary modifications, and stool softeners are part of a comprehensive bowel program.

Mental Retardation

Mild cognitive delays are frequently associated with muscular dystrophy. Some children may demonstrate more severe mental retardation.

Additional Resources

To learn more about muscular dystrophy, you may wish to contact the organizations listed in the Appendix.

SEIZURE DISORDERS

Description

Seizures are relatively common disorders of infants and children. They are generally more common in the first two years of life than in later years (Whaley & Wong, 1987). Seizures can, however, be present into adulthood.

Seizures are an indication that the brain is undergoing sudden, abnormal bursts of electrical activity. They are manifested in a variety of symptoms ranging from muscular twitching to a convulsion affecting the entire body. For example, the affected area may be limited to a small area and result in symptoms such as a stiffening of one arm, or may affect most of the brain as in a generalized convulsion. Seizures may also be characterized by alterations in consciousness, feeling, behavior, sensation, and autonomic function. After the seizure, the child's brain returns to its normal functioning.

Epilepsy refers to seizures which occur repeatedly in an otherwise healthy child or when a child has a medical condition that is associated with seizure activity (Epilepsy Foundation of America, 1985).

Causes

There are many causes of seizures. With most seizures, the exact cause is unknown. The seizure may be caused by a time limited condition such as an extremely high temperature or a sudden blow to the head. In these situations, the seizures go away after the temperature drops or the body recovers. These children may never have a recurrence of seizure activity. They do not have epilepsy.

Other children have a genetic tendency toward seizures. This tendency may be related to lowered seizure thresholds, congenital defects, or familial electroencephalographic abnormalities (unusual brain waves).

Still other children may have seizures that are acquired rather than genetic. These seizures are the result of brain injury during the prenatal, perinatal or post-natal period. Trauma, insufficient oxygen, infections, biochemical imbalances, or exposure to toxins can produce seizure activity.

Factors that contribute to seizure activity include fatigue, stress, unusual excitement, illness, and physiological changes (hormonal and metabolic).

Seizure Types

While the physiological mechanisms are similar, seizures are classified according to how much of the brain is involved at the beginning of the episode. The International Classification of Epileptic Seizures divides seizures into two categories: partial and generalized.

Partial Seizures

Partial seizures begin locally. They are further divided into simple partial, complex partial, and partial seizures (secondarily generalized [Jacksonian]).

Simple partial seizures   These seizures are focal since they are limited to one area of the brain. They result in localized motor, sensory, psychological or autonomic symptoms, or a combination. The child generally does not lose consciousness.

In some children, the seizure is motoric. One of the most common motor actions is an aversive seizure in which the child's eyes and/or head may turn to one side. The arm on that side may be extended and fingers clenched.

In other children, the symptoms are sensory. The child may experience distorted sounds, smells, or feelings. Numbness, tingling, or prickling may occur.

Complex partial seizures (also called psychomotor or temporal lobe) While originally thought to originate in the years from five through adolescence, enhanced diagnostic equipment such as video-telemetry is documenting that this type of seizure may be seen as early as infancy.

This type of seizure has an associated impairment of consciousness. It is preceded by an aura, or vague premonition. Since the temporal lobe which controls sensation is involved, the aura may involve the sense of smell, taste, sound, or emotions. Some children hear voices. These symptoms may precede the seizure by as much as 24 hours.

The seizure itself is characterized by a sequence of automatic behavior in which consciousness is lost or clouded (Epilepsy Foundation of America, 1987). It may begin with a blank stare. Automatic behavior such as chewing, lip smacking, buttoning and unbuttoning clothing, or picking at clothing occur. Some children even attempt to take off their clothes.

Consciousness is generally impaired. Children often appear to be drugged or to be sleepwalking. Although alert, the children are unaware of their surroundings. They may mumble or appear confused. Their actions are clumsy and nondirected. They may appear frightened and try to run. Often they struggle or flail when someone tries to restrain them. Observers may confuse these seizures with emotional or psychiatric disturbance, or drug abuse.

Complex partial seizures last a few minutes, but confusion may persist for hours. The child does not remember what happened during the seizure. Symptoms of complex partial seizures may vary among children. However, the pattern is the same for all seizures in a particular child.

Partial seizure (secondarily generalized [Jacksonian])   This type of seizure is characterized by a partial seizure with impaired consciousness, that then becomes generalized. Under this classification, the seizure starts in one part of the body, usually with localized jerking in the arm, leg, or face. It cannot be stopped but the child remains awake and alert. Later, the seizure may become more generalized. This type of seizure is often associated with underlying structural pathology. Medical evaluation for possible underlying causes is indicated.

Generalized Seizures

The second category of seizures is generalized. These seizures usually affect both sides of the body. They do not start in a localized area, and there is impaired consciousness. These seizures are divided into generalized tonic-clonic, absense, myoclonic jerks, febrile, neonatal, and myoclonic-akinetic.

Generalized tonic-clonic seizures (formerly known as grand mal)   Generalized tonic-clonic seizures may begin anytime after the newborn and infancy period. This seizure is a generalized convulsion that involves the entire body. It is generally what is envisioned when the term epilepsy is used.

The seizure may be preceded by a period of unusual irritability, anxiety, or confusion. The child may experience strange, vague sensations before the seizure begins. The seizure may start with a sudden cry. The child loses consciousness and falls to the ground. The child's muscles become rigid (tonic phase) and then start jerking rhythmically (clonic phase). Breathing is often shallow or labored. The child may temporarily stop breathing, and the skin may become bluish. The child may lose bowel or bladder control for a few minutes.

The seizure usually lasts less than 5 minutes. Normal breathing starts again. The seizure may be followed by confusion, fatigue, headache or drowsiness, and deep sleep. After 1 to 2 hours, the child will return to full consciousness and resume normal activities. The child will have no memory of the event. These seizures may occur several times a day, or as infrequently as once a year.

Most children who have seizures, even generalized tonic-clonic seizures, have normal intelligence. They do not seem to suffer brain damage as a result of the seizures. Most children can be well controlled on anticonvulsant medication and eventually outgrow the seizure activity.

Absence seizures (formerly known as petit mal)   This type of seizure is very common and usually begins when the child is 4 to 10 years of age. (It rarely occurs before 3 years of age or after 20 years.) The seizure is characterized by a period of unresponsiveness lasting less than 10 seconds. It is often described as blank staring spells. The seizure begins and ends abruptly. Rapid blinking or chewing movements may occur. No tonic-clonic movements or drowsiness take place. The child is not aware of the seizure or the environment during the seizure. Upon completion of the seizure, the child is fully aware of the surroundings once again.

Since these seizures may occur up to 100 times a day, a child may unknowingly be unaware of many activities in the environment. If these seizures are undetected in the school setting, learning problems may occur. No first aid is necessary, but the child should be referred to the physician for an evaluation when the seizure is noted for the first time. Many children outgrow this condition, although some children have (or eventually develop) generalized seizures.

Myoclonic jerks (formerly known as infantile spasms)   This type of seizure usually begins between 3 months and 2 years of age. The seizures are clusters of quick, sudden, bilateral, symmetrical muscle contractions. Infantile spasms may take the form of sudden jack-knifing forward of the body (hence the lay term "jackknife epilepsy" or "salaam seizures").

If the child is sitting up, the head may fall forward and the arms may flex forward. If the infant is lying down, the knees will be drawn up and the arms and head flexed forward. This jack-knifing may occur five to ten times in a row for 30 seconds, and reoccur periodically throughout the day. As the child gets older, the convulsions may continue as described or may combine with more generalized tonic-clonic movements.

Infantile seizures can be associated with several conditions: Tay-Sachs disease; metabolic diseases such as phenylketonuria; Down syndrome; tuberous sclerosis; or infections such as meningitis. Sometimes, the cause is unknown.

No first aid is indicated. However, the child should be referred to a physician for a medical evaluation when the seizures are noted for the first time. If effective treatment is started early, future seizures may be controlled. However, many children with infantile spasms, especially those with uncontrolled seizures, have later developmental delays.

Febrile seizures   This type of seizure occurs most often in the period from 3 months to 4 years of age. It is rarely noted before 6 months of age or after 5 years of age. A febrile seizure is characterized by a generalized convulsion which occurs when the infant has a high temperature (usually above 104 degrees Fahrenheit). The cause of the fever is generally a relatively common childhood condition such as an ear infection, a viral infection, or a rash. The seizure lasts about 10 minutes and involves tonic-clonic movements of all extremities. It is short-lived and does not reoccur.

There is a lot of medical controversy regarding the advisability of treating febrile seizures with anticonvulsant medication. However, the majority of children who have one febrile seizure do not have another, even if they are not on anticonvulsant medication.

Febrile seizures are often preventable by careful monitoring of temperatures and the use of a tepid water bath (never alcohol) to bring down a high temperature.

Neonatal seizures   Seizures that occur in the neonatal (newborn) period typically involve shaking of one or two extremities. The infant may engage in breath-holding and may lose consciousness. The eyes may move rhythmically or stare (Batshaw & Perret, 1986). Infants may not have generalized seizure activity, if their neurological system is too immature for such coordinated activity.

Newborn seizures may be the result of brain malformation or abnormality leading to mental retardation or cerebral palsy. Seizures may also result from brain damage caused by too little oxygen during the perinatal period. Intraventricular hemorrhages (bleeding within the ventricles of the brain) lead to stroke-like symptoms and may contribute to seizure activity. Seizures associated with these severe disorders have a poor prognosis and are difficult to control.

Some newborn seizures are caused by temporary imbalances in the levels of calcium or sugar in the blood. Hypocalcemia (low blood calcium) or hypoglycemia (low blood sugar) may result. If these conditions are recognized early and treated promptly, there may be little or no residual effects.

Myoclonic-akinetic seizures   These myoclonic seizures should not be confused with the myoclonic jerks (infantile spasms) discussed previously. These seizures are characterized by brief involuntary jerking of all or part of the body, without loss of consciousness.

Akinetic seizures are characterized by loss of movement. During a seizure, the child may suddenly collapse and fall. After a few seconds, the child recovers fully and continues usual activities. These seizures are often referred to as "drop attacks."

These two types of seizures are often related to neurological damage or degenerative disease. Many of these children also have conditions that cause mental retardation.

Myoclonic-akinetic seizures are difficult to diagnose, since they are often confused with clumsiness. Due to the severe, underlying disease process, they are often difficult to control with anticonvulsant medications.

Detection

Careful documentation of seizure activity and frequency is the basis for a clinical diagnosis. Brain wave tests (electroencephalogram or EEG) are usually done. However, seizure activity does not always show up on an EEG, so this is not the sole determining diagnostic test.

Health Problems

Associated Conditions

Seizures are also associated with diseases such as cerebral palsy, hydrocephalus, and mental retardation. If the child has these underlying problems, they must be considered when treating the seizures.

Side Effects of Medications

Seizures are treated with anticonvulsant medications. These conditions control the seizures but do not cure them. Because these medicines are very powerful, they may cause some medical side effects. Most commonly, anticonvulsants cause drowsiness and gastrointestinal distress, such as nausea and vomiting. Dilantin, a commonly used anticonvulsant, causes gum irritation. Good oral hygiene is imperative to prevent serious complications.

Be sure to check with the child's doctor to learn the side effects that may occur from any medications the child is taking. Notify the parents and the physician if these side effects are noted. Also notify the parents and the physician when seizures occur. Many times, a child's growth results in the need for increased medication doses to assure continued seizure control.

Learning Disabilities

Children who have frequent episodes involving loss of consciousness may experience gaps in learning. They may also have difficulty following classroom instructions. As a result, they are at increased risk for experiencing later learning problems.

Behavior Problems

Many children with epilepsy demonstrate behavior problems. These are usually related to the disorderly nature of the world and frustration resulting from lack of control. It is critical that professionals address issues related to self-concept and psychosocial adjustment. The fact that seizure activity can occur at any time makes it more difficult to adjust to epilepsy than to some other chronic diseases.

Additional Resources

Refer to Chapter 9 for a discussion of emergency treatment of continuous generalized seizures (status epilepticus) and to Chapter 6 for a discussion of monitoring and documentation of seizures. To learn more about seizures, you may wish to contact the organizations listed in the Appendix.

SPINA BIFIDA

Description

Spina bifida means cleft spine. It is an incomplete closure of the spinal column. It can involve the skin, spinal column, and spinal cord. There are three types, each with a different degree of severity. (See Figure 3-3 for pictures of the types of spina bifida.)

Spina Bifida Occulta

This is the most common and least involved type of spina bifida. In spina bifida occulta, there is generally an opening in one or more vertebrae (bones) of the spinal column. There is no damage to the spinal cord and no obvious lump on the back. This type of spina bifida usually causes few if any symptoms. In fact, many people are not aware they have the condition.

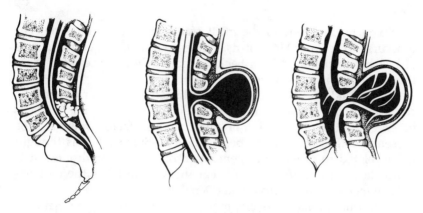

A. Spina Bifida Occulta   B. Meningocele   C. Myleomeningocele

Figure 3-3. Three types of spina bifida. Reproduced by permission of Paul H. Brookes Publishing Company, P.O. Box 10624, Baltimore, MD 21285-0624 and G. Gordon Williamson, Ph.D., O.T.R.

Meningocele

This is the least common type of spina bifida. In meningocele, the meninges, or protective covering around the spinal cord, does not form properly. Instead, the meninges is pushed out through an opening in the vertebrae and into a sac called a "meningocele." This sac protrudes out somewhere along the spinal column. The sac under the skin can vary from the size of a nut to the size of a grapefruit. The meningocele can usually be corrected surgically, with little or no nerve damage. Since the spinal cord is not affected, there is no spinal cord damage.

Myelomeningocele

This is the most severe type of spina bifida and occurs more frequently than the meningocele form. In myelomeningocele, there are openings in both the vertebrae and the spinal cord. There is also a sac which pouches out at some place along the spinal column; this sac may contain meninges, spinal fluid, and spinal cord. Some or all of these nerves are not properly connected to the spinal cord and/or brain. This sac has little or no skin protection, so infection is a very serious potential threat. Surgery is generally scheduled within 48 hours of birth. The surgery can remove the sac and reduce the danger of infection. However, it will not cure any paralysis or lack of feeling.

Cause

Spina bifida is one of the most common types of birth defects. It occurs in 1 to 2 per 1,000 births. Incidence is higher in ethnic groups of Welsh, Scottish, and Irish backgrounds, although the reasons for this difference is not known.

Spina bifida is believed to be a multifactorially inherited genetic condition. This means that the tendency to have spina bifida is inherited, but the interaction of environmental factors must also be present for the condition to be manifested. Spina bifida is thought to be related to other more general chromosomal syndromes. It is also believed to occur when a pregnant woman takes the anticonvulsive medication, valproic acid (Depakene).

In normal prenatal development, the neural tube or spinal cord (myelo) forms into a straight column covered first by membranes (meningo) and later by the spine. Spina bifida is classified as a neural tube defect. This type of defect means there has been a disruption in the normal development of neural tube closure and the formation of the spinal column over the neural tube (spinal cord). The continuum of neural tube defects varies from spina bifida occulta to protrusion of the brain (encephalocele) or spinal cord (myelomeningocele) to open or absent brain development (anencephaly).

A neural tube defect can often be identified prenatally. Maternal alpha-fetoprotein screening can be used to detect abnormal levels of the protein in the mother's blood. Because alpha-fetoprotein is found in high concentration in spinal fluid, abnormally high levels usually indicate leakage of spinal fluid into the amniotic fluid, and ultimately into the mother's blood stream. Because other conditions such as twins and fetal death may also result in high alpha-fetoprotein levels, confirmatory ultrasound testing is often recommended. Amniocentesis can also be used to determine levels of alpha-fetoprotein in the amniotic fluid. These tests are not 100% accurate, but have increased the percentage of open neural tube defects identified during pregnancy.

Common Health Problems

Spina bifida is not a progressive disease. However, children are at great risk for the development of a variety of medical complications. The prognosis and medical course of a child with spina bifida depends to a great degree on the location and extent of involvement of the spinal nerves. Some very involved infants do not live, but most children do. Early surgical correction of the defect is usually necessary to prevent generalized infection (sepsis) or infection of the brain (meningitis).

Children with myelomeningocele are in need of comprehensive, interdisciplinary support, including child and family support and measures designed to increase socialization and self-esteem. Preventive and early therapeutic measures aimed at medical consequences of the condition will greatly enhance later abilities and quality of life. The establishment of good health and self-care habits is critical to the prevention of untoward complications.

Hydrocephalus

Because the spinal cord is the system through which fluid is drained from the brain, spina bifida also affects the normal exchange of cerebral-spinal fluid. Problems with cerebral-spinal fluid exchange occur in 70% to 90% of all children with spina bifida. If the fluid cannot drain off, extra fluid accumulates in the brain, and a condition known as hydrocephalus occurs. A drain (shunt) can be used to equalize fluid flow. Shunt failure or repeated infections can result in brain damage. (Refer to section on Hydrocephalus in this chapter for further information.)

Poor Muscle Control

Because there is so much nerve involvement in myelomeningocele, there is usually a lot of nerve damage to the area below the involved part of the spinal cord. The spinal cord is divided into four parts: cervical, thoracic, lumbar, and sacral (Williamson, 1987). Figure 3-4 illustrates these spinal regions.

The higher the location of the defect on the spinal column, the greater the severity and extent of involvement will be. Thus, involvement of the brain and/or cervical (neck) vertebrae may affect the face and all limbs. If the lumbar area is involved, ambulation is affected. If the sacral area is involved, there may be problems in digestive motility, and bowel and bladder dysfunction.

Depending on the part of the spinal column that is affected, the child may not be able to ambulate. In many children, ambulation is possible with the use of bracing or special adaptive equipment or devices. Physical therapy is particularly important in preserving range of motion and weight-bearing abilities. Children with limited weight-bearing ability may be more prone to fractures of the lower extremities.

Scoliosis

Structural defects of the spine and poor muscle control can result in problems with the alignment of the spinal column. Curvature of

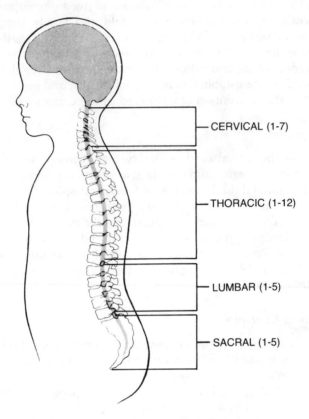

CERVICAL (1-7)

THORACIC (1-12)

LUMBAR (1-5)

SACRAL (1-5)

Figure 3-4. Regions of the spine. Reprinted from *Medical aspects of developmental disabilities in children birth to three* by J.A. Blackman, p. 201, with permission of Aspen Publishers, Inc., copyright 1990.

the spine (scoliosis) is a frequent result. Such malalignment may make maintenance of proper postural alignment difficult. Improper posture can also contribute to the development of pressure points on the skin and cause internal pressure on critical internal organs. Orthopedic care and possible surgery may be indicated to correct deformities.

Skin Breakdown

Lack of sensation may contribute to the development of skin problems. Since the child is not able to feel pressure, positions may not be changed frequently. As a result, skin surfaces may be subjected to pressure for long periods of time. Circulation is impaired, and the areas of affected skin may begin to break down. A similar process occurs if the child is unable to feel injury or damage due to contact with irritating substances, such as urine or feces. Initial signs are redness and swelling. Indications for referral to a physician are as follows: a sore that does not heal or is getting larger; a yellowish, thick discharge from the area; or a sore that is open and draining.

Sometimes, a medication is prescribed to combat an infection, but the child has an allergic reaction. Overall rash, localized skin redness, burning and itching sensations (if the child has feeling in the area) may indicate an allergic reaction. Stop the medication and call the physician immediately.

It is much easier to prevent skin breakdown than to cure it. Thorough cleaning (especially of skin areas that have come in contract with urine or feces) is critical. Frequent position change and gentle massage increases blood circulation and impedes the development of skin problems.

Protection from skin injury is also important. Protect the child against cuts or bumps as much as possible. Removal of sharp objects in the immediate environment will help, as will consistent use of clothes and shoes as additional protection. Help the child to avoid temperature extremes in the weather or in the objects in the environment. Lack of sensation will mean that the child may not avoid an extremely hot or cold object that someone else would instinctively pull away from. Carefully assess skin areas that may come in contact with adaptive appliances or wheelchairs to detect areas of friction and rubbing. Avoid tight fitting adaptive appliances, shoes, or clothes.

Bladder Problems

Because the nerves responsible for bladder control are located in the lower part of the spinal cord, most children with myelomeningocele have bladder problems. There are two types of bladder anomalies. The first is a flaccid bladder due to poor muscle tone. Children with this problem are often not able to tell when the bladder is full. Hence, they do not feel the urge to urinate. Because they are not able to fully empty their bladder, they often require regularly scheduled procedures such as clean intermittent catheterization to remove urine from the bladder. (Refer to Chapter 6 for a discussion of clean intermittent catheterization.)

Irritable or spastic bladders also present a problem. Children with this condition find it difficult to control the urinary sphincter. They suffer from incomplete emptying, with an accumulation of pressure in the kidney. The presence of residual urine in the bladder, following incomplete emptying, predisposes the bladder and kidney to infection. It also contributes to urinary dribbling and incontinence (lack of control). Poor management of urinary problems can result in serious kidney damage.

Bladder problems also predispose the child to urinary tract infections. Adequate fluid intake, hygiene practices, and careful observation for signs and symptoms of infection are important to prevent the development of serious infection. Medications are often used to improve bladder storage and continence, as well as to treat infections.

Bowel Problems

The nerves responsible for bowel control are also located in the lower spine. Children with myelomeningocele may also have problems with bowel control. Hypomotility (low level of movement of the intestines) contributes to problems with constipation, bowel blockage, and bowel incontinence (lack of control). Nutritional management and bowel training programs at school are critical.

Obesity

Lack of mobility and poor self-esteem contribute to problems with obesity. Obesity may aggravate the development of pressure sores and skin breakdown. Nutritional management and active physical therapy programs are important.

Learning Problems

Most children with spina bifida have normal intelligence. In fact, many children are often placed in regular classrooms. However, some children, especially those who have suffered from hydrocephalus, may demonstrate learning problems, eye-hand coordination problems, or some degree of attention disorder. Children who have experienced brain damage as a result of hydrocephalus may be irritable, demanding, emotionally labile, and easily frustrated.

Additional Resources

To learn more about spina bifida, you may wish to contact the organizations listed in the Appendix.

BIBLIOGRAPHY

American Academy of Pediatrics, Committee on Infectious Diseases. (1987). Health guidelines for the attendance in day-care and foster care settings of children infected with Human Immunodeficiency Virus. *Pediatrics, 79,* 466-471.

American Academy of Pediatrics. (1989). *Report of the Committee on Infectious Diseases* (21st ed.). Elk Grove, IL: Author.

American Academy of Pediatrics, Task Force on Pediatric AIDS. (1988). Pediatric guidelines for infection control of Human Immunodeficiency Virus (Acquired Immunodeficiency Virus) in hospitals, medical offices, schools and other settings. *Pediatrics, 82,* 801-807.

Black, J., & Jones, L. (1988). HIV infection: Educational programs and policies for school personnel. *Journal of School Health, 58,* 317-322.

Blackman, J. (1984). *Medical aspects of developmental disabilities in children birth to three.* Rockville, MD: Aspen.

Bresnahan, K., Brooks, C., & Zuckerman, B. (1991). Prenatal cocaine use: Impact of infants and mothers. *Pediatric Nursing, 17*(2), 123-129.

Centers for Disease Control. (1987). Classification system for Human Immunodeficiency Virus (HIV) infection in children under 13 years of age. *Morbidity and Mortality Weekly Report, 36,* 225-236.

Centers for Disease Control. (1988). Update: Universal precautions for prevention of transmission of Human Immunodeficiency Virus, Hepatitis B Virus, and other bloodborne pathogens in health care settings. *Journal of the American Medical Association, 260,* 462-464.

Centers for Disease Control. (1989). Guidelines for prevention of transmission of Human Immunodeficiency Virus and Hepatitis B Virus to health-care and public safety workers. *Morbidity and Mortality Weekly Report, 38,* 1-37.

Centers for Disease Control. (1990). Estimates of HIV prevalence and projected AIDS cases: Summary of a workshop, October 31-November 1, 1989. *Morbidity and Mortality Weekly Report, 39,* 110-119.

Crocker, A., & Cohen, H. (1988, August). *Guidelines on developmental services for children and adults with HIV infection.* Baltimore: American Association of University Affiliated Programs for Persons with Developmental Disabilities.

Fischl, M., Dickinson, G., Scott, G., Klimas, N., Fletcher, M., & Parks, W. (1987). Evaluation of heterosexual partners, children and household contacts with adults with AIDS. *Journal of the American Medical Association, 257,* 640-644.

Gerberding, J., Bryant-LeBlanc, C., Nelson, K., Moss, A., Osmond, D., Chambers, H., Carlson, J., Drew, W., Levy, J., & Sande, M. (1987, July). Risk of transmitting the Human Immunodeficiency Virus, Cytomegalovirus, and Hepatitis B Virus to health care workers exposed to patients with AIDS or AIDS-related conditions. *The Journal of Infectious Disease, 156*(1), 1-8.

Graff, J., Ault, M., Guess, D., Taylor, M., & Thompson, B. (1990). *Health care for students with disabilities: An illustrated medical guide for the classroom.* Baltimore: Paul H. Brookes.

Jackson, P. (1990). Primary health needs of children with hydrocephalus. *Journal of Pediatric Health Care, 4*(2), 59-71.

Lifson, A. (1988). Do alternate modes for transmission of Human Immunodeficiency Virus exist? *Journal of the American Medical Association, 259,* 1353-1358.

Lozes, M. (1988). Bladder and bowel management for children with myelomeningocele. *Infants and Young Children, 1*(1), 52-62.

March of Dimes Birth Defects Foundation. (Undated). *Down syndrome.* White Plains, NY: Author.

Miola, E. (1987). Down syndrome: Update for practitioners. *Pediatric Nursing, 13*(4), 233-237.

National Down Syndrome Society. (Undated). *Fact sheet.* New York: Author.

National Down Syndrome Society. (Undated). *Questions and answers about Down syndrome.* New York: Author.

National Information Center for Handicapped Children and Youth. (Undated). *Down syndrome.* Washington, DC: Author.

Pueschel, S., Tingey, C., Rynders, J., Crocker, A., & Cruther, D. (Eds.). (1987). *New perspectives on Down syndrome.* Baltimore: Paul H. Brookes.

Roberts, C. (1988). Bowel management in spina bifida: Perspectives and issues. *Barrow Neurological Institute Quarterly, 4*(4), 37-41.

Rogers, M., White, C., Sanders, R., Schable, C., Kesell, T., Wasserman, R., Bellanti, J., Peters, S., & Wray, B. (1990). Lack of transmission of Human Immunodeficiency Virus from infected children to their household contacts. *Pediatrics, 85,* 210-214.

Shandling, B., & Gilmour, R. (1987). The enema continence catheter in spina bifida: Successful bowel management. *Journal of Pediatric Surgery, 22*(3), 271-273.

Van Dyke, D. (1989). Medical problems in infants and young children with Down syndrome: Implications for early services. *Infants and Young Children, 1,* 39-50.

Voeltz, L. (1980). Children's attitudes toward handicapped peers. *American Journal of Mental Deficiency, 84,* 455-464.

Wolraich, M. (1984). Spina bifida. In J. Blackman (Ed.), *Medical aspects of developmental disabilities in children: Birth to three.* Rockville, MD: Aspen.

4

WORKING
COLLABORATIVELY
WITH
THE FAMILY

It is impossible to care for a child with special health care needs without working collaboratively with that child's family. Although professionals may be very involved for a period of months or even years, the family's relationship with the child remains constant for a lifetime. Family members have the ultimate responsibility for decisions that will affect the life of the child with special health care needs. It is the responsibility of all professionals to help the family by practicing family centered care. This approach is based on family support for natural caregiving and decision-making roles; it is implemented by building on the unique strengths of individuals and families (Brewer, McPherson, Magrab, & Hutchins, 1989; Shelton, Jeppson, & Johnson, 1987). Family centered care is particularly beneficial to children who suffer from an ongoing health problem (Perrin, 1985). To practice family centered care, professionals must first understand family responses to living with a child with special needs, factors that influence adaptation, common family concerns, and recommended professional strategies for helping to meet family concerns.

FAMILY RESPONSES

Imagine that you are leaving work one day, in a hurry to meet someone at a predetermined time in a local park. As you get to your car, you discover that you cannot locate your car keys. Your first response is one of almost panic. "I cannot find my keys! Where are they?" Your continued search is unproductive. Your next response will probably be one of denial. "I could not have lost my keys. I never lose them. I had them with me this morning. This cannot be happening to me."

Finally, you acknowledge that indeed your keys are nowhere to be found. By now, your colleagues have all gone home and you must call someone to come to get you. At this point, guilt and anger may begin. "I cannot believe I have lost my keys. That was certainly stupid. Everyone else has gone home now, and I must wait alone."

As you wait, anxiety may increase. "How am I going to get word to my friend that I will be late. Will my friend worry? Am I going to be safe here alone until my rescuer arrives? I bet all my colleagues are already home preparing dinner by now."

You resign yourself to the fact that there is little that can be done to change the situation, and you sit down on a nearby rock to await your ride. As you wait, you begin to modify your plans for the evening, so it will be enjoyable after all.

Although this exact situation may not have happened to you, you can probably identify with many of the feelings that occurred. They are normal responses to unexpected situations. While losing car keys can in no way be equated with learning that your eagerly awaited newborn has special health care needs, it does serve as a basis for understanding the process a family undergoes as it learns of the diagnosis and attempts to adapt to its implications (I. Hernandez, personal communication, June 26, 1991). This process is common to all families, regardless of the specific diagnosis.

Shock

Families do not plan to have a child with special health care needs. The situation usually takes them by surprise and affects all members of the family. It is understandable that an unexpected diagnosis is generally followed by a period of shock. The family, who had eagerly awaited the birth of a perfectly normal child, is told that the child has special health care needs. Families relate that this stage is similar to "walking around in a daze, sure that this situation is not really happening" (I. Hernandez, personal communication, June 26, 1991).

Denial

The next stage is denial of the diagnosis. The period of denial is especially evident if the condition is not immediately obvious. Examples are a child with a severe neurological problem which does not become outwardly noticeable until 2 years of age, or mental retardation in a child who has no external characteristics. Families in denial often go from one physician to another, seeking a different or more acceptable diagnosis. In their denial state, they sometimes misinterpret treatment regimens by thinking, "If I follow all the professional recommendations, my child will recover and be totally normal."

This stage is a necessary one for parents and professionals must allow time for parents to work through it. Denial becomes problematic when it prevents the family from following through on necessary medications or treatments. Denial may also contribute to unrealistic parental expectations of the child's abilities. In these situations, intervention may be beneficial to help the family through this stage.

Sadness, Anger, Guilt, and Anxiety

The next stage is characterized by sadness, anger, guilt, and anxiety. A mother writes "I was so mad! Not just at the fact that I had a child with a disability—I was mad at everything . . . the weather, friends, doctors (really mad at doctors), our health insurance carrier (this anger was totally justified) and the dog (and I don't even own one)!" (Johnson, 1991, p. 46).

During this stage, guilt and self accusation may be apparent. Parents generally anticipate nothing less than the perfect child (Simons, 1985). The process of grieving the "loss of the perfect child" often results in guilt and related alterations in self-esteem. The parents (as a couple) may blame each other, with subsequent additional stress on their relationship.

To cope with these feelings of guilt, families may become overprotective. They may feel that no one else is qualified to care for their child. This lack of trust may extend to the spouse or to professionals.

It may contribute to arbitrary decisions regarding school attendance or participation in classroom activities.

Parents may also demonstrate overprotectiveness by avoiding discipline. It is easy to attribute undesirable behaviors such as temper tantrums to the child's illness; however, many times these activities are age-related rather than a part of the diagnosis (Association for the Care of Children's Health, 1989). In an effort to protect the child from possible further discomfort, the parents may thwart opportunities for increased independence in self-care and lifestyle decisions (Urbano, 1987). As a result, the child may miss many of the normal experiences of childhood.

When family members experience guilt, they may also have difficulty sharing the diagnosis with others. When parents feel the condition reflects a defect in themselves, a lowered level of self-esteem may develop. As a result, family members may withdraw socially.

Parents frequently acknowledge that guilt also affects their participation in normal health promotion activities, such as recreation. They may have difficulty accepting their right to have fun or participate in activities without their child. Parents may experience guilt for actually enjoying themselves.

Anger at health professionals who made an unpopular diagnosis or were unable to make an early diagnosis is frequently noted. Anxiety may occur as the family begins to consider the long-term impact of the condition, the lack of a definite diagnosis or the uncertainty of ongoing care when the parents are too old to continue. Professionals must be aware of this anger, and realize that it is not a reflection of their skills.

Parents report that sadness, anger, anxiety, guilt, and frustration never really disappear (I. Hernandez, Personal Communication, June 26, 1991; Johnson, 1991). The feelings may be rekindled as they see a healthy child walking when theirs cannot, or as they hear another parent complain about relatively minor inconveniences of parenting. Chronic sorrow is especially strong at holidays such as birthdays and Christmas. It is also exacerbated at key transition points, such as the time the child might ordinarily start to walk or talk, enter school, enter puberty or graduate from high school. Sadness, anger, and anxiety are also felt strongly if the child undergoes frequent hospitalizations or experiences significant surgery. Fear of the unexpected becomes particularly significant, because family members have already experienced the unexpected and know such events can happen to them (I. Hernandez, personal communication, June 26, 1991).

Chronic feelings of sadness persist as families recognize that life will never be the same. Unexpected demands and expectations may contribute to role confusion and frustration. Although their life may be rewarding and their child may be very loved, parents realize life will not be as originally planned, through no choice of their own (I. Hernandez, personal communication, June 26, 1991).

Siblings are also affected by the addition of a child with special needs. They experience reductions in available parental time, changes in lifestyle and routine, and frequently additional caregiving responsibilities for their affected sibling. It should be emphasized, however, that siblings do not necessarily experience higher rates of psychological impairment or symptoms than other children (Breslau, Weitzman, & Messenger, 1981). Sibling response is strongly influenced by the degree of adaptation of the family unit as a whole. In fact, parents have reported that siblings of a child with a disability are often more sympathetic, understanding, independent, and communicative than other children (Pinyerd, 1983).

Adaptation and Reorganization

The final stage is adaptation. At this time, the family develops a new sense of balance in the family system (Gallo, 1991). The family demonstrates a realistic acceptance of the diagnosis. The child is integrated into the family and considered to bring positive attributes to the family setting. Families become increasingly involved in activities shared with other families of similar age and background.

These activities support assumptions that families facing hardships develop basic strengths designed to foster growth and protect against disruptions (McCubbin & Patterson, 1983). During such crises, families benefit from and contribute to community resources and relationships (McCubbin & McCubbin, 1987).

While earlier research hypothesized the inevitable serious negative consequences of having a child with a chronic condition, more recent literature documents a range of success in adaptation (Walker, Epstein, Taylor, Crocker, & Tuttle, 1989). Successful family adaptation requires substantial changes in roles, routines, and family interactions (Benoliel, 1975). When families are able to adapt and reorganize, they generally experience improved family strength and additional skills to handle future crises (McCubbin & Patterson, 1983). Poor adaptation, however, may result in continuing crises or spousal divorce (McCubbin & Patterson, 1983).

Adaptation as a Dynamic Process

Although families agree that these stages are valid, they hasten to note that they are dynamic. Progression may not be made from one stage to another in sequence. Indeed, families frequently move back and forth between stages and may share elements of several stages simultaneously (I. Hernandez, personal communication, June 26, 1991). Thus, it is critical to be sensitive to the needs of the family at the present and to accept frequent changes in family response.

FACTORS THAT INFLUENCE ADAPTATION

Responses to illness vary dramatically, even with children who have the same diagnosis. The ease with which families adapt can be positively or negatively influenced by many factors.

Perceptions

One's perception of a situation is even more important than the reality of that situation. This is true when a child has special health care needs. Thus, it is necessary to explore how the family perceives a child's needs.

Cause

Part of the initial adjustment to an illness is the search for a reason for its occurrence. Scientific logic generally provides a cause for illness in the form of an organism or pathological dysfunction. However, people often consciously or unconsciously attribute the occurrence of illness and disability to other causes. For example, some perceive illness to be caused by negative thoughts, "unacceptable behavior," or witchcraft. Others view illness as a test of their religious convictions or a challenge to their role as family protector. Frequently, the imagined cause is strongly influenced by culture.

Preventability

The perceived degree of preventability is closely related to the imagined cause (Moulton, 1984). Guilt implies acceptance of a degree of control. If the family member feels control over the prevention or alteration of a condition, that individual is more likely to feel increased guilt. This helps to explain increased evidence of guilt when a genetic condition or avoidable injury occurs.

Illness and Its Impact

One's perception of an illness and its impact is based on the previous knowledge of an illness. For example, an infant has just been diagnosed as having Down syndrome. Assume the parents know another family with a child with Down syndrome. If the other family has adapted well to their child and feel that, while difficult at times, their situation has also brought much joy to their lives, the new parents would probably not perceive the diagnosis as catastrophic. If, however, the other family had faced repeated hospitalizations and surgeries, and ultimately experienced divorce, the new parents may feel their family's future is threatened. This perceived impact of an illness is a more critical predictor of future adaptation than the actual severity of the condition.

Value of the Illness

Adaption to illness is also influenced by the perceived value of the condition. For example, if illness is viewed as a matter of shame and dishonor, families may have difficulty acknowledging the condition and seeking outside assistance for its management. If the illness is perceived as a challenge that can be effectively met with a unified family effort, the adverse consequences will be minimized.

Imagined Cure

Cure is related to treatment. If the family feels the only viable cure is metaphysical, they may not be receptive to traditional medical management. If the family feels the condition is the result of witchcraft, they may not be receptive to medication and physical therapies. Thus, professionals must include a family's perceived cure strategy into the proposed treatment regimen.

Developmental Stage

The developmental stages of family members relates to the ages of family members, developmental task expectations, demands, resources and prior experiences. For example, young teenage parents who are grappling with their own identities and the establishment of family and career, view a child's illness from a very different perspective than older parents.

The developmental stage of the child when an illness is first diagnosed is also important. Many times it is easier for a family to deal with a disability in a newborn than to cope with an older child who experiences a sudden devastating illness or accident.

Individual Characteristics

Because the family is the sum of its individual members, characteristics of each person in the family can positively or negatively contribute to family strength. Characteristics such as intelligence and knowledge and skills regarding the child's condition are important factors in the child's care. So are the family members' general health knowledge, individual physical and mental health, adaptability, self-esteem, and organizational abilities.

Family Resources

The pre-existing roles and relationships within a family can provide the basis for future strengths or conflict. Variables such as family organization, routines, distribution of responsibility, cohesion and support, communication styles, adaptability, and problem-solving abilities should be considered (Gallo, 1991). These family relationships and the place of the child in the family set the basis for modification of roles and responsibilities.

The sibling of a child with special health care needs is a special family resource. Siblings want to be an active participant in family decisions, but do not want to become overloaded with responsibility. Siblings share many of the same concerns as parents, and go through the same stages of adaptation. Siblings may be automatically considered to be another caregiver, regardless of age. They often become confused with conflicts between the role of family member and caregiver, just as parents do. Thus, professionals must be sure to involve siblings in all stages of assessment and care planning as well as be cognizant of their special needs (M. Sutton, personal communication, July 15, 1991).

Family resources also include financial resources. A child with special health care needs generates unexpected financial requirements for medical care and therapies. While governmental financial assistance exists on a limited basis, it may be available only to families with lower incomes. If a parent must quit a previous job to provide child care, money will become more limited. Obviously, families that are fortunate to have increased financial means broaden their alternatives for medical care, therapies, respite, and recreation.

Probably one of the most important family resources to consider is coping styles. Family response to previous crises is a good predictor of the degree of success in coping with the current situation. Families with a high degree of adaptation frequently use an increased number of coping strategies. Thus, if one strategy is not effective, others may be substituted. Successful coping strategies are often associated with increased self confidence and enhanced self-concepts.

Community Supports

In addition to family relationships and resources, members benefit from extended family and community supports. Knowledge of available community agencies, and the willingness to utilize these organizations, can provide additional supports. These resources may include professional health care services, nonrestrictive school environments, social support networks and responsive government policies (Gallo, 1991).

Cultural Expectations

Many roles and relationships are influenced by the family's culture. In many cultures, a child is not considered to be an equal member of the family unit. In some cultures, the child is seen as insurance for old age, so a child with a disability is viewed as a threat to the family's future security. Culture will also influence the degree of acceptance of recommended treatments and therapies, as well as family roles in decision-making and caregiving. Cultural values, myths and realities, familial roles, and religious beliefs will influence the family's perception of the problem and pattern of seeking help.

Caregiving Demands

The daily demands for care are perhaps more important than the diagnosis, because two children with the same diagnosis may need very different care. Caregiving responsibilities are closely related to increases in financial stressors, physical and emotional fatigue, and need for respite. Anxiety often occurs when family members must assume responsibility for complex medical treatments. Families also have increased responsibilities to assure that school activities and therapies are continued in the home setting.

Concurrent Stressors

Understandably, it is easier to adapt to the child with special health care needs when everything else affecting the family is going smoothly. When families face financial crises, transportation difficulties, marital conflict or maladaptive behavioral responses, such as abuse of drugs and alcohol, the situation is only exacerbated. As such external stressors build up, coping with the medical needs of the child becomes increasingly difficult.

COMMON FAMILY CONCERNS

Researchers have documented that childhood illness and disability is often associated with increased family stress (Clements, Copeland, & Loftus, 1990; Gallo, 1991; Kohrman, 1990; Walker, Epstein, Taylor, Crocker, & Tuttle, 1989). Sources of stress relate to family concerns in several areas.

Changes Within the Family

Family adaptation necessitates many changes. Expectations and plans are modified as the family begins to make a place for the child. Roles and responsibilities are modified or expanded to compensate for the additional caregiving and organizational responsibilities. The complexity of caregiving routines frequently decreases spontaneous family outings, especially those involving only the parents.

Increased Caregiving Responsibilities

Most children with special health care needs require additional care. Not only are medical treatments, medications, and therapies required, but even feeding, bathing and dietary management become more complex. These activities are frequently accompanied by family questions such as, "Am I doing this procedure correctly? Will other people care for my child correctly? What will the long-term consequences of medications and treatments be?"

Caregiving becomes even more complex if the family assumes responsibility for care-coordination. Not only are care-coordination activities time consuming, they are very frustrating. This frustration is often increased because of the natural emotional involvement of the family.

Loss of Privacy

As parents assume increasing responsibility for care, they find themselves involved with an increasing number of professionals. While well-meaning, these professionals are generally attempting to gather additional information about the family's strengths and needs. This increase in the number of interviews and home visits by professionals results in a decrease in family privacy.

Increased Need for Support

Parenting a child with special health care needs requires an extensive expenditure of physical and emotional energy. The situation seems even more draining with the realization that the requirements are never-ending (I. Hernandez, personal communication, June 26, 1991).

At a time when family members need to draw energy from the emotional support of others, they may feel isolated from family and friends. Sometimes, this feeling of isolation is a result of the lack of time and energy. At other times, it is the result of the withdrawal of others who are struggling with their own adjustments to the situation.

Psychological support from friends and family and emotional support from parent-to-parent groups help to ease the unnecessary drain of emotional reserves. Such contacts also help to show family members how to compensate. They are invaluable in helping the family feel they are not alone, that others are experiencing the same feelings, and that they are normal (M. Sutton, personal communication, July 15, 1991). Community respite programs provide additional relief by providing a much needed break from constant caregiving responsibilities.

Uncertainty About the Future

Parents often express concern about the future. They are often concerned about the future abilities of their child and the management of the child's care, especially when the parents die. Siblings also worry about their responsibilities once the parents are gone, and the impact it will have on their own lives (M. Sutton, personal communication, July 15, 1991). Family members also express anxiety regarding their abilities to respond appropriately in the case of an emergency.

Information Needs

Families have many information needs. Some are related to the diagnosis, treatment, and implications of the diagnosis on daily care. This includes strategies for disciplining the child; normalizing the child's environment and activities; coping with siblings; explaining the condition to others; and problem solving. To provide comprehensive care, families need information about community programs and services, resources for modification of housing, legal assistance, transportation, insurance, obligations of the educational systems, and legal rights of the family. Unfortunately, education for families often excludes important information about routine parenting issues common to all children, especially content related to growth and development sequences and accident prevention.

Financial Support

The need for additional information extends to finances. Families incur many out-of-pocket expenses for travel, parking, physician services, and medication (Walker, Epstein, Taylor, Crocker, & Tuttle, 1989). Loss of time and increased frustration often accompany the search for information regarding financial resources and methods of accessing financial supports.

Time Management

Being a parent is time-consuming at best. When the parent must incorporate time for additional procedures, doctor's visits and medication administration, along with time allocated for the rest of the family, time management becomes critical.

Role Conflict

Many parents report conflict between the roles of parent and caregiver. This conflict is especially evident if the parent must balance the parental role of pain alleviator with the role of the caregiver responsible for performing painful procedures (Kohrman, 1990). Role conflict also occurs if the child is hospitalized or has full-time nursing care in the home. Parents report feeling a need to be sure all care is scrutinized and coordinated among various disciplines and specialists.

Coordination Between Home and School

Parents frequently voice concerns regarding the need to access educational testing and placement quickly. They are also concerned about the effective coordination of therapies and learning activities between home and school. Mainstreaming and balancing medical care and education are related areas of interest.

Parent/Professional Relationships

Families frequently express frustration about their relationships with professionals. They feel professionals do not treat the family as an equal member of the team. Appointments are scheduled at the convenience of the professional, not the family. The professional often does not really listen to family concerns or family input about diagnosis or intervention plans. Professionals seem to be reluctant to provide complete information, answer questions or describe situations without medical jargon. These actions may be viewed by the family as a lack of empathy and respect on the part of the professional, or a lack of understanding about the requirements of home care (Stonestreet, Johnston, & Acton, 1991).

RECOMMENDED PROFESSIONAL STRATEGIES

To assist families in addressing their concerns, professionals must adopt a family-centered approach to care. This necessitates viewing the family as an equal member on the interdisciplinary team, and a lead partner in care-coordination. Based on this perspective, several specific professional strategies are recommended.

Respect the Family as a Unique Unit

Although professionals voice acceptance of families as equals, subtle actions such as not listening to the family, lack of acceptance of varying values and priorities, and withholding of full information demonstrate that much progress is needed. Parents must be acknowledged as the experts about their child and the child's care. Well-intentioned professionals must become increasingly sensitized to their behaviors and the needs of families.

Part of respect is the acknowledgment of the need for privacy. As comprehensive family assessments are becoming more commonly used, professionals must not lose direction. Professionals must all remember that the goal is "to understand what families want for themselves and their children and what they need from professionals in order to achieve those aspirations" (Bailey, 1991, p. 27).

Listen to Families

Families and professionals both benefit when parents relay information about their children. It is especially important for families to share their joys, fears, and concerns during crises periods, such as acute illness, hospitalization or key developmental transitions. Professionals should also listen to family ideas and reactions and include them in all aspects of care planning and coordination. Because family members know the child better than anyone else does, they are more prepared to individualize care.

Active listening involves establishing a comfortable safe environment, reading body language, and acknowledging family feelings. It also includes recognizing the family's strengths and needs, as well as their goals and priorities in life. These techniques are effective in further opening lines of communication (Stonestreet, Johnston, & Acton, 1991).

*Accept Variability in Family Interest, Coping Styles,
and Degree of Involvement*

Families are made of individuals first, families second, and families
with a child with special health care needs third. They vary just
as all families do. Their reactions are strongly influenced by their
perceptions of the situation and appropriate methods of dealing with
it. Professionals must allow the family to be the determiner of decisions and interventions.

Additionally, professionals must be sensitive to the family's current position in the grieving process and acknowledge the dynamic
nature of adaptation. Monsen (1986) has suggested that the family/
professional relationship evolves, depending on the family's status
in the adaptation process; professional styles should change accordingly. For example, during the period of early diagnosis, families
may need more information and professional caregiving. Later, as
the family becomes more comfortable in caregiving activities, the
professional should function in a more equal role. When families
are able to progress to leadership positions in parent groups and
advocacy organizations, the professional should become a consultant
(Monsen, 1986).

*Include Families as Equal Partners in all Activities Related to
Needs Assessment, Planning, and Evaluation*

Professionals should ask families what they view as their
strengths and the areas in which they would like assistance. They
need to acknowledge and build upon family strengths. The child's
likes and dislikes and family schedules should be considered in the
development of intervention plans. Additionally, the professional
should demonstrate an open, flexible attitude and a willingness to
work out responsive interventions. During the assessment and intervention phases, the professional should maintain verbal contact
with the family, discuss current progress, and work out modifications
together (I. Hernandez, personal communication, June 26, 1991).
When it is time for a periodic evaluation of progress, the professional
should ask the families how interventions worked for them, and
modify interventions accordingly. Remember that while professionals plan for short-term goals, families determine success in terms
of outcomes (Stonestreet, Johnston, & Acton, 1991). The professional
should fully discuss expectations to avoid misunderstandings.

Provide Full and Clear Information to Families

Family members will serve as the guide to what information
they need and when it is needed. If you do not have all the infor-

mation, admit it. Families state they would rather be told, "This is what we know at present" or "With some children . . . , with other children . . . . We do not know specifically how your child will do" (I. Hernandez, personal communication, June 26, 1991).

If the prognosis is poor, families ask professionals to soften the shock. Rather than saying "Johnny cannot live longer than 6 months", say "There is a strong possibility that Johnny may not live beyond 6 months. We will need to see how he does." This allows the family to focus on living day to day, but does not take away all hope (I. Hernandez, personal communication, June 26, 1991).

Information should be based on the gamut of family needs. It should include not only information about the condition and its management, but also resources and rights. Focus on problem solving, open family communication, expansion of the repertoire of coping strategies, and health promotion/relaxation behaviors. The family should be provided with the opportunity to practice procedural skills, including emergency management. Also, prepare family members to deal with the questions and reactions of others in the family and community. Often adverse reactions from strangers are based on lack of understanding. Family members are in an ideal position to enlighten the public.

Include anticipatory guidance in teaching. Discuss anticipated behaviors that accompany an upcoming developmental stage and possible methods of handling issues related to those behaviors. Such advance warning prepares families for previously unexpected events and allows them to develop strategies for dealing with these situations. Such techniques also contribute to enhanced feelings of self-control and self-esteem.

Assist The Family in Accessing Support Networks

These networks may be related to health care delivery, social services, transportation, legal services, housing, finances or parent-to-parent support. Regardless of the content, support networks reduce frustration and isolation. They are critical adjuncts to family empowerment, for they assist families in realizing they are not alone.

Encourage Normalization

Assist the family and child to have as normal a life experience as possible. Encourage the family to respect the child as a unique and special individual. Since many children with special health needs have developmental delays, base activities on developmental rather than chronological age or size. Encourage activities that promote exploration, self-acceptance, and enhanced self-esteem. Life experiences increase individual independence, productivity, and integration into the community. It is day-to-day experiences that enhance the quality of life for us all.

Final Strategy

Working collaboratively with families takes time. To quote Stonestreet and her colleagues (1991, p. 46), "Sometimes things that take time, save time." But, when such collaborative relationships exist, everyone benefits. So, be patient, honest, and open. Let the family know you are available to work jointly with them to provide an improved life for their child.

BIBLIOGRAPHY

Florida Department of Education. (1990). *Family functioning: The impact of a child with special needs: Model of interdisciplinary training for children with handicaps, module 4.* Tallahassee, FL: Author.

Holvoet, J., & Helmstetter, E. (1989). *Medical problems of students with special needs: A guide for educators.* Boston: College-Hill Press.

5

FROM REFERRAL
TO
PLACEMENT

The entry of a child with special health care needs into the school setting requires extensive preparation to assure a smooth transition. The process frequently starts with a contact from the parent or the hospital discharge team, but can be initiated by anyone.

At the initial contact with the school, general information, including the child's name, address, phone number, date of birth, and diagnosis is obtained. At this time, information can be obtained about the parent's health and medical concerns, the child's typical day (including routine schedules, necessary medical and health procedures), and the child's current level of functioning. A decision must then be made regarding placement in a regular or a specialized classroom. If a regular classroom cannot be modified to meet the child's needs, interdisciplinary assessment and planning must be initiated.

The process begins with the family's comprehensive orientation, including delineation of rights and responsibilities. The parents should be asked to identify physicians and representatives of other community agencies who may have important background information. School professionals should request parental release of information as well as their assistance in obtaining relevant records. Recent information must be included, since the child's medical needs may change very quickly.

INTERDISCIPLINARY ASSESSMENT

The interdisciplinary team represents many different professions. Its goals are to work collaboratively with the family to assess the strengths and needs of the child and family; jointly develop a plan to meet those needs; determine responsibilities to complete planned interventions; and evaluate the degree of goal attainment.

The interdisciplinary approach facilitates the view of the child and the complex child/family relationship from a system-oriented perspective. The family is conceptualized as a series of dynamic, inter-related components in which the child affects the family, as well as the family members influencing the child. In addition to a system-wide assessment, the child is evaluated in terms of psychological, cognitive, physical, social, behavioral, nutritional, sociocultural, environmental, and developmental status. At the same time, the family's functioning, as well as formal and informal support systems, is assessed.

Review of Existing Records

The process begins with a review of prior collaborative data. This information is gathered from physician's records, prior evaluations, and the files of other community agencies. Such records provide valuable background data and can often mean avoidance of unnecessary duplications in testing. Since families are understandably sensitive about personal and confidential information, always respect the laws and ethics of confidentiality.

While this is a logical and important first step, it is often difficult to obtain discriminate, accurate, and relevant histories and medical information. Even when obtained, many records are incomplete or outdated. If the child is currently hospitalized or recently discharged, the hospital team may be an invaluable resource for the successful search for current, useful information.

The hospital-based interdisciplinary team is convened to make arrangements for subsequent discharge. The team's first task is to determine the feasibility of the child's discharge. Considerations include the stability of the child's medical condition, the family's readiness and interest in providing care, and the suitability of environmental and community supports. At times, a home visit may have been included to determine the suitability of the child's home as a support for care.

The hospital discharge team is responsible for planning a home-based plan of care and assuring that the family has been taught critical home care procedures. In some areas, members of the discharge team are available to train personnel in procedures that may be required during the school day.

Identification of Strengths and Areas of Need

Once available background information and additional interdisciplinary assessments has been gathered, the interdisciplinary team can identify additional areas needing testing.

The results of all records and current testing are synthesized. Then the team, with active participation from the family, is ready to address strengths and needs in the following key areas.

1. The child's diagnosis (including description of the condition; severity; associated medical problems; and contraindications for school attendance);
2. Special procedures/treatments that may be necessary during the school day (and their side effects);
3. Special medications that must be given during the school day (including type of medication; action; implications for teaching; side effects; danger signs; and route of administration);
4. Special nutritional requirements (including nasogastric or gastrostomy tube requirements);
5. Special adaptive appliances or equipment that the child may need to supplement daily activities;
6. Independence in self-care activities, and potential for further independence;
7. Urinary or bowel problems, if any;
8. Special precautions or limitations, if any;
9. Educational implications (including possible limitations in: vision; hearing; speech/language; mobility; vitality; positioning; attention and activity levels; cognitive limitation due to diagnosis or medication; special infection control measures; need for more frequent bathroom breaks, snacks or rest periods; modifications for physical education; potential for involvement in classroom activities; anticipated school absence);
10. Emergency measures and precautions (including warning signs and symptoms; probability of emergency; appropriate

responses; emergency contacts; plans for fire and natural disaster);

11. Current resources (i.e., electrical specifications; personnel available to perform procedures; classroom modifications; educational/communication equipment needs);

12. Additional resources needed (including additional personnel; specific training; environmental modifications such as temperature control; environmental hazards; running water; refrigeration; additional electrical requirements; treatment or storage areas; transportation modifications);

13. Any family factors that would support or negatively influence the child's care.

DEVELOPMENT OF AN INDIVIDUALIZED FAMILY SERVICE PLAN

Based on the findings of the interdisciplinary assessment, an Individualized Family Service Plan is developed. As with other stages of the process, the development of the Individualized Family Service Plan is developed with the active participation of the family. While the format and content varies slightly, it generally includes the following:

1. Statement of the infant or child's present level of physical, cognitive, language, speech, and social development;

2. Current level of self-help skills;

3. State of the family's strengths and needs, as related to the enhancement of the child's growth and development;

4. Statement of the major outcomes expected to be achieved, with criteria, procedures and timelines;

5. Statement of the specific intervention services necessary to meet the identified needs, including the frequency, intensity, and anticipated method of service delivery. This includes day-to-day care and emergency plans as well as delineation of responsibilities for various facets of implementation as well as appropriate classroom placement;

6. Projected dates of initiation and anticipated duration of services;

7. Identification of the care-coordinator;

8. Plan for periodic review with parents and re-evaluation, as indicated. Review should always be made following hospitalization or change in treatment regimes, to be sure intervention is congruent with current medical status.

IMPLEMENTATION OF THE INDIVIDUALIZED FAMILY SERVICE PLAN

Naturally, the assessment and planning phases serve as the basis for subsequent intervention. Functional abilities take precedence over diagnosis, since there is much variation of abilities within diagnostic categories. For many children, ability to benefit from educational placement is dependent on the extent to which the illness or condition interferes with daily functioning and learning (Walker, 1984). Thus, intervention alternatives must take into account the child's needs on a daily basis. The child and family members are usually the best source of information regarding the feasibility and effectiveness of the interventions.

Orientation/Training

An essential step in implementation is to prepare staff for the child's arrival. If the child has an unfamiliar or complex condition, the staff may have many questions. Frequently these questions revolve around the condition itself and its implications for education, modifications which must be met to accommodate the child's needs, responsibilities for any medications or procedures, communicability of the condition and potential liability.

These and related questions are best handled through carefully planned orientation sessions, conducted on two levels. First, a general orientation for school personnel and other students. Depending on the situation, this orientation may range from a brief introduction that a new student will be joining the class to a more in-depth discussion of special needs of the child.

The second level of preparation is a more detailed training session for direct care providers. These sessions may include written materials as well as presentations. If medication administration or medical procedures are involved, individualized training must be conducted. These sessions should be completed prior to the child's admission into the school setting, to assure appropriate safety and supervision. (Refer to Chapter 6 to learn more about physician and family permissions and guidelines for specific training and procedures and to Chapter 9 for emergency preparedness).

Simultaneously, the child and family, and the child's physician should be oriented to the school. Training and orientation programs should include the family in all aspects of planning and implementation, to assure family involvement and continuity between home and school.

Specific orientation of the child to the school will depend on the individual situation. Some children adapt more easily if they enter the school for only short periods of time at first; others are comfortable with a full schedule from the start. Arrangements can be made collaboratively with the family and school, and modified as appropriate for the child.

Provision of Adequate Resources

While adequate resources necessary to meet the child's needs were identified as part of the interdisciplinary planning phase, the resources must now be obtained and adequate functioning assured. Resources may include increased staffing to handle more time-consuming services; additional personnel properly trained and supervised to perform required procedures; standards and policies to guide future activities (if not already available); more comprehensive emergency plans and procedures; and increased communication among school, family, and physician regarding daily management issues.

Implementation of the Plan

The intervention plan must be implemented in a timely manner, to avoid unnecessary stress for the child and family. Careful coordination of the plan is necessary to enhance the quality and continuity of care. This approach reduces fragmentation and duplication of services, and facilitates access.

EVALUATION

The ongoing suitability of the plan, and the degree to which it promotes goal attainment must be evaluated periodically by both the family and the professionals. This is particularly important if the child's medical condition changes dramatically, such as occurs with hospitalizations or surgery. Careful planning and monitoring are critical to assure the child with special health care needs is able to access the educational system quickly, and that planned intervention services are consistently supportive to the child and family.

BIBLIOGRAPHY

Billings, J., Schrag, J., Kirsch, G., Brattain, J., Peck, J., & Maire, J. (1989). *Medically fragile technical assistance manual.* Olympia, WA: State Superintendent of Public Instruction.

Caldwell, T. (Ed). (1990). Hospital Outreach: Making a difference in the education of a child. *Step by Step, V*(9), 1-3.

Caldwell, T., Todaro, A., & Gates, A. (Eds). *Community provider's guide: An information outline for working with children with special health needs.* New Orleans, LA: Children's Hospital.

Haynie, M., Porter, S., & Palfrey, J. (1989). *Children assisted by mechanical technology in educational settings: Guidelines for care.* Boston: Children's Hospital.

Holvoet, J., & Helmstetter, E. (1989). *Medical problems of students with special needs: A guide for educators.* Boston: College-Hill Press.

McGonigel, M., & Garland, C. (1988). The individualized family service plan and the early intervention team: Team and family issues and recommended practices. *Infants and Young Children, 1*(1), 10-21.

Pearl, L., Brown, W., & Myers, M. (1990). Transition from neonatal intensive care unit: Putting it all together in the community. *Infants and Young Children. 3*(1), 31-50.

6

MANAGING THE CHILD'S HEALTH PROBLEMS

An increasing number of children with special health needs are now being integrated into early intervention and school settings. Court decisions mandate that increasingly complex "related services" are provided in the school setting. Many different disciplines share responsibility for managing these health problems. Management strategies fall into three categories: general supervision of a child's health problem; medication administration; and performance of health related procedures.

Activities related to general supervision fall within normal responsibilities and do not require additional written permissions from the parent and physician. Medication administration and performance of actual procedures require the development and implementation of policies and procedures to safeguard both the child and the professional. This chapter contains discussions of management strategies, suggestions for appropriate policies and procedures, and general information regarding some of the most frequently requested services. The chapter will, of necessity, be more detailed and procedurally oriented than other sections of this text.

The material presented in this chapter provides guidelines to assist school personnel in establishing safe environments for children with special health care needs. However, the reader is cautioned to develop customized plans for an individual child in collaboration with the child's own physician. The reader is further cautioned that these guidelines provide general information. Professionals should explore state legal guidelines for practice in their state before beginning care. Professionals who will be actively involved in health care should receive individualized training, including ongoing supervision and support, from the child's physician or the school nurse prior to performing the procedures independently.

GENERAL SUPERVISION OF A CHILD'S HEALTH CONDITION

Health problems require ongoing observation on the part of all professionals who interact with the child with special health care needs. The purpose of these observations is the early detection of unusual behaviors or responses which may indicate a complication or medical emergency. If possible complications are noted, the professional's role is to notify the parents and the physician and to document the observations and actions in writing. If a medical emergency is noted, the professional's role is to take emergency action, including notification of the emergency medical services system team, and the initiation of cardiopulmonary resuscitation and other first aid measures, as indicated. (Refer to Chapter 9 for discussion of emergency measures.)

Although professionals routinely make observations of children in their care, there are several conditions that warrant special monitoring and attention.

Seizure Management

Seizure activity may vary dramatically in appearance (refer to Chapter 3 for a complete discussion of seizures). Seizures also vary in the effect on the child and the classroom management required (Epilepsy Foundation of America, 1987). Professionals share many health-related responsibilities: (1) administration of medications (usually anticonvulsants) that will help to control seizures; (2) first aid when a seizure occurs; (3) recognition and referral of emergency situations requiring immediate medical evaluation; (4) documentation of seizure activity; and (5) communication with parents, physician, and other children in the classroom.

Medications to Control Seizure Activity

The seizure activity of most children with epilepsy can be controlled through daily medication. Other children may receive partial control with medication. For a small percentage of children, a medication or combination of medications, is still insufficient to totally control seizure activity.

Different medications are used to manage specific types of seizure activity. The dose will vary according to the seizure behaviors the child demonstrates, as well as variables such as the child's age, weight, metabolism, and individual response to the drug. The type and amount of anticonvulsants may have to be modified frequently to adjust to changes in the child's growth and health status.

Anticonvulsant medications are generally safe, but many of them have side effects. Drugs commonly used with children include Phenobarbital, Dilantin, Zarontin, and Depakene. Side effects from these drugs may include the following: drowsiness; hyperactivity; loss of muscular coordination; confusion; nausea and loss of appetite; swelling of the gums; slurred speech; tremors; and difficulty sleeping. These symptoms, if they do occur, are generally mild. The physician tries to balance the benefits of the medicine against its disadvantages. Because school personnel see the child more frequently than the physician does, their observations are important and should be recorded and reported to the parents and physician.

Teachers or other school personnel may be asked to administer anticonvulsant medications during the school day, to keep optimal amounts of the medication in the child's blood stream at all times. Since these medications are powerful, care must be taken that they are administered properly. (Refer to the part of this chapter that discusses medication administration in the school.)

First Aid When A Seizure Occurs

When a child with seizures is enrolled in the school, the parents should be contacted regarding the usual seizure activity demonstrated by the child and the responses that are usually necessary. Explore school policies to determine organizational guidelines for appropriate responses.

Seizures are not generally an emergency situation. In fact, some seizure activity may go unnoticed. Once a seizure has started, no attempt should be made to stop it. Be sure the child is protected from injury from objects in the environment.

Absence seizures   This type of seizure is often described as blank staring spells. There is nothing you can do during this type of seizure. Document its occurrence, and report it to the school nurse or parent. If you are the teacher, be sure the child is not missing important material due to frequent absence seizures. If this does occur, additional instruction or review is indicated.

Simple partial seizures   This type of seizure is characterized by localized motor, sensory, psychological or autonomic symptoms or a combination. Since senses are often distorted during these seizures, the child may need some special comfort and reassurance.

Complex partial seizures   These seizures are characterized by loss or distortion of consciousness. Amnesia and increased anxiety are often present. In response to this type of seizure, avoid stopping or restraining behaviors. Move harmful things out of the child's path. Use a calm voice and slow movements while the child is having a seizure. Provide comfort and reassurance.

Generalized seizures   This term includes generalized tonic-clonic, myoclonic jerks, febrile seizures, neonatal seizures, and myoclonic-akinetic seizures. During generalized seizures, part or all of the child's body will stiffen, the child may cry out and fall unconsciousness, and the body may jerk repeatedly. The child may also lose bowel and bladder control. The child does not feel any pain and does not remember what happened during the seizure. Generalized seizures are frightening to the observer and lead to a feeling of helplessness, but there are some basic things you can do.

If a generalized seizure does occur, do the following:

1. Keep calm; reassure other staff and children that the child will be fine; have someone else care for the other children while you attend to the child with a seizure.
2. If the child is sitting or standing, lower the child to the floor.
3. Loosen the clothing around the child's neck. Put something soft under the child's head. If possible, turn the child's head to the side, to enable saliva to drain from the mouth and to help breathing.
4. Do not try to restrain the child's activity, but, remove hard, sharp or hot objects from the child's immediate area.
5. *Do not force anything between the child's teeth.* This response is a common misconception and can be dangerous. Do not try to hold the child's tongue, or force the mouth open. The child will not swallow the tongue, but it could block the airway. To prevent blockage, turn the child's head to the side.
6. The child may stop breathing briefly or turn slightly blue during the seizure.
7. After the seizure, examine the child to be sure other injuries did not occur. The child may need assistance in getting cleaned if bowel and bladder control were lost. (Keep extra

clean clothing at school in case it is needed.) The child will also probably be very tired. Let the child rest if desired. If the child is not too tired, classroom activity can be resumed.

8. Do not offer anything to drink until the child is fully awake.

Recognition and Referral of Emergency Situations

The average seizure (even a generalized convulsion) is not a medical emergency and resolves without problems. *Immediate medical attention is recommended if:*

1. The child has a seizure and there is no known history or cause. Medical evaluation is indicated to determine the cause;
2. If consciousness does not return after the seizure, or if the child had a head injury during the seizure. The possibility of head injury should be considered in the presence of the following symptoms: difficulty in arousal after 20 minutes; vomiting; visual problems; persistent headache; unconsciousness; or dilated or unequal pupils.
3. The child has a seizure in the water.
4. If the seizures last longer than 5 minutes, or if the child goes from one seizure to another without regaining consciousness between episodes. Although this rarely happens, *it is a medical emergency and the emergency medical services team should be called immediately.* This response will permit the appropriate emergency care in a timely manner.
5. If breathing does not resume spontaneously, start emergency cardiopulmonary resuscitation (see Chapter 9).

Documentation of Seizure Activity

Because seizures generally happen at school or in the home, the child's physician does not usually have an opportunity to observe them. Consequently, the documentation of the seizure activity is important to help the physician determine future action.

Documentation should include the following: the date; time; length of seizure (timed by using a clock, if possible); description of what happened; child's behavior afterwards, and what was done afterwards. (See Figure 6-1 for an example.)

Communication with Parents, Physician, and Other Children in the Classroom

If the child has frequent seizure activity and has sustained no injury in the current seizure, a phone call or note to the parents

Figure 6-1.   Sample seizure log.

NAME OF CHILD:

DATE:

TIME SEIZURE STARTED: TIME SEIZURE ENDED:

WHAT WAS THE CHILD'S BEHAVIOR DURING THE SEIZURE?
(Any warning signs?; how did seizure start?; what parts of the body were
involved?; what was the sequence of involvement; was consciousness lost?;
did the child lose bowel and/or bladder control?)

WHAT WAS THE CHILD'S BEHAVIOR AFTER THE SEIZURE?

DID THE CHILD RECEIVE ANY INJURIES DURING THE SEIZURE? IF
SO, WHAT WAS DONE TO TREAT THE INJURIES AND WHAT WERE
THE EFFECTS OF THAT TREATMENT?

This form should be filed in the child's school record. Copies should be
sent to the parents and the child's physician. Seizure activity should be
noted on a flow sheet or calendar to document patterns. All forms should
be reviewed periodically to determine if the frequency or nature of seizure
activity has changed. Report changes to the parents and physician.

is sufficient. Be sure to alert the parents if the seizures seem to change
in frequency or nature. If the child's behavior is different in any
way, suggest that the child's physician be contacted to see if medical
evaluation is indicated. If this is the child's first seizure or if the
situation warranted immediate medical attention (see Recognition
and Referral of Emergency Situations section), refer the parents for
an immediate medical evaluation. Share your observations of the
event with the physician to facilitate diagnosis and management.
Of course, if the seizure involves a true medical emergency, contact
the emergency team first, then the parents.

Other staff and children in the school setting may become concerned when seizures occur. This is true even for infants and toddlers
who are developmentally delayed. Although they may not really
understand what is going on, they are frequently aware of the
emotional environment and unusual activity. Explain that their friend
will be fine soon, and there is no reason to be afraid. If the children
are able to understand, give more complete explanations.

Monitoring a Shunt (Hydrocephalus)

Hydrocephalus and the placement of shunts to control hydrocephalus were discussed in Chapter 3. Monitoring and related documentation of the child with a shunt is often the responsibility of
school-based personnel. Since there is no actual contact with the

shunt, monitoring consists of identifying child behaviors that may indicate increasing intracranial pressure. It is helpful to establish a routine procedure for documenting student behavior such as general level of activity, as well as awareness of and response to the environment. In some areas, sequential head circumferences are measured and recorded. Variations from normal patterns over time may indicate a developing problem.

Infection

Infection of a shunt is a major complication. It occurs most commonly in the first 2 to 4 months following shunt placement or revision (replacement). Early symptoms may be subtle, with later symptoms becoming more noticeable. Symptoms include the following:

1. Nausea and vomiting;
2. Headaches;
3. Lethargy or irritability;
4. Lack of appetite;
5. Fever;
6. Redness or swelling along the surgical site (incision) or tubing;
7. Abdominal pain (in the case of a ventriculoperitoneal shunt);
8. Rubbing of the ear on the side of the shunt (in infants).

Fluid Buildup

Even with a shunt in place, fluid buildup may occur if the tube is disconnected internally, if there is leakage, or if there is a kink or blockage in the tubing. Such conditions may contribute to cerebrospinal fluid buildup in the ventricles. Warning signs include the following:

1. Headache;
2. Nausea and vomiting;
3. Irritability or restlessness (sometimes with a high pitched cry in infants);
4. Personality or behavioral change;
5. Change in alertness or orientation to the environment (including drowsiness or lethargy);
6. Seizures;
7. Bulging fontanel (if soft spot is still open);
8. Abnormally small pupils that respond slowly to light. (More severe problems are dilated and fixed pupils, especially if associated with increased pulse and irregular breathing. If untreated, death may follow.)

If you notice any of the symptoms listed, the parent and physician should be notified and your observations documented in writing. However, avoid over-reacting. Children with shunts also get colds and the flu. These conditions can also cause headaches, nausea, and vomiting. The presence of these symptoms in a child with a shunt should include a pediatric evaluation as any other child would receive, prior to extensive neurological workups to determine the possibility of shunt failure.

A word of caution. Some shunts have a reservoir or pump which can be seen as a small button under the skin at the point of insertion (usually behind the ear). In the past, some parents and professionals were instructed to "pump the shunt" to test for proper functioning of the shunt. This practice is now controversial.

The valve in the pump is designed to be activated when ventricular pressure reaches certain levels. Otherwise, it does not need to work. If the shunt is "pumped" unnecessarily, the pressure in the ventricles may drop to dangerously low levels. For this reason, pumping the shunt is not advised unless specifically directed to do so, and procedurally instructed by the child's physician.

MEDICATION ADMINISTRATION

In many states, one of the most common health related responsibilities of school personnel is administration of medication during the school day. The administration of medication is a potentially dangerous activity, because mistakes could have devastating consequences. Caution must be taken to assure that the proper medication is given by the appropriate route, at the correct time, and to the correct child.

Why Are Medications Administered in the School Setting?

Medications are administered for many reasons. Some medications are given to cure symptoms or reduce pain. For example, Acetaminophen is given to reduce an elevated temperature and reduce pain. Some medications, such as antibiotics, are given temporarily to cure an illness. Medications may also be given to prevent complications or assist normal physiological functioning. Other medications are given to replace compounds normally found in the body.

At times, medications may be given only once or a few times. In other situations, such as with seizure medication, the child may take the medicine for a lifetime. Many medicines must be given at regularly scheduled times throughout the day, to assure that there is a constant level of medicine in the blood at all times.

Who Decides What Medications A Child Should Receive?

Giving medications to a child as part of one's professional responsibilities is quite different from giving medicines to your own child. For one thing, you cannot legally decide when to give a medication, or to actually administer any medication, even Acetaminophen, without appropriate permission from the physician and the parent.

Physician Permission to Give Medications

Physician written permission should be received prior to giving any prescription or over-the-counter medication. This can be accomplished by supplying the physician with a written form detailing the following: child's name, address, and birthdate; name and dose of medication; reason for medication; special instructions; beginning and ending dates for administration in the school setting; precautions; side effects (including ones which should be reported to the physician); the physician's name, address, phone number, signature; and the date of the prescription. (See Figure 6-2 for sample physician permission form.)

It is the responsibility of the person administering the medication to consult with the physician for further clarification when the physician order (permission) is not clear, or if there are any questions concerning the appropriateness of the order or its execution in the school setting.

Parental Permission to Administer Medications

In addition to physician authorization to administer medications, parental permission must also be obtained. Permission forms should contain the child's name, date of birth, and address; medication name, dosage and hours of administration; special instructions or precautions; beginning and ending dates for school administration of medication; name and phone number of physician; authorization to communicate with the physician and to give medication in the school; release of claim of liability; parental agreement to notify the school of any changes in medication or dosage; parental agreement to provide medication to the school and obtain refills as indicated; parental name, address, phone number, signature and date. (See Figure 6-3 for sample parental permission form.)

Safety Precautions

Training Regarding Medication Administration

Prior to giving any medication, the school professional should be trained by a registered nurse or physician. The training should include medication use and side effects, storage and administration procedures, emergency responses, recording, and actual supervision of the medication administration process. The instructor should document in writing that you have been trained, components of the training, and that you successfully demonstrated safe and accurate medication administration. These statements will provide legal verification that you were appropriately trained.

Because these comments help to transfer some legal responsibility to the instructor, the registered nurse or physician may wish to periodically re-evaluate competency. This re-evaluation is to your advantage and should be encouraged. Document periodic supervision of your ability to administer medication safely and accurately. This action will serve to document ongoing competency to perform these activities.

Figure 6-2.   Sample physician permission form.

MEDICATION ADMINISTRATION

This form must be completed for all prescription and over-the-counter medications to be given in the school setting. Medications should be administered at school only when failure to receive such medication could jeopardize the health of the child.

This form should be revised as needed after each acute illness or hospitalization. The maximum period of authorization is for one year.

Child's Name: _____ Child's Date of Birth _____
Child's Address: _____

The above child is under my medical supervision. I have prescribed the following medication.

Name of Medication: _____ Dose: _____
Times of Administration: _____
Special Instructions or Precautions: _____

Reason for Medication: _____
Possible Side Effects: _____

Course of Action If These Side Effects Should Occur (Including Identification of Side Effects Which Should Be Reported to the Physician):

Beginning and Ending Dates for Administration in the School

_____   _____
(Beginning Date)   (Ending Date)

Physician's Name: _____ Address: _____
Phone Number: _____
Physician's Signature: _____ Date of Prescription: _____

Figure 6-3. Sample parental permission form.

MEDICATIONS

This form must be completed for all prescription and over-the-counter medications to be given in the school setting. Medications should be administered at school only when failure to receive such medication could jeopardize the health of the child. This form should be revised as needed after each acute illness or hospitalization. The maximum period of authorization is for one year.

Child's Name: _____ Child's Date of Birth _____

Child's Address: _____

Name of Medication: _____ Dose: _____

Times of Administration: _____

Special Instructions or Precautions: _____

Beginning Date for Administration: _____

Ending Date: _____

Physician's Name: _____

Physician's Phone Number: _____

I hereby request that my child be given the above medication while in school and away from school for official activities. I understand that the medication may be given by trained non-medical personnel. I give my permission for appropriate personnel to communicate with my child's physician in matters related to medication and health supervision. I understand that medication administration will not begin until physician and parental permission forms are on file, and personnel have been properly trained. I understand that the law provides that there shall be no liability for civil damages as a result of the administration of such medication where the person administering such medication acts as an ordinarily reasonable and prudent person would under the same or similar circumstances.

I understand that I must notify the school of any changes in my child's condition, medication or dosage. I further understand that I am responsible for ensuring the medication safely arrives at school and for getting refills of the medication as indicated.

Parent's Name: _____

Parent's Phone Number:_____

Parent's Address: _____

_____   _____
(Parent's Signature)   (Date)

Note: This form should be completed by parent or legal guardian.

Medication Storage

It is the parent's responsibility to assure that medication is purchased and transported to the school. It is the responsibility of the school to provide safe storage of the medication, proper administration and monitoring, and safe return back to the parent for administration during "out of school" hours.

A medication should be received and stored in its original container, with the original label. This helps to assure the correct contents of the container. When at school, the medication should be stored in the original container in a locked area, not in the child's bag where it can be found by other children. If the medication needs to be refrigerated, a locked box can be placed in the refrigerator to provide safe storage.

It is the parent's responsibility to refill medication prescriptions. However, many parents have difficulty planning ahead. It is helpful for school personnel to send a note home to the parents reminding them that it is almost time to refill the prescription. Careful planning avoids unnecessary disruptions on medication regimes and the harmful side effects that can accompany abrupt termination of certain medications.

Prevention of Medication Errors

There are many types of medication errors (mistakes). Giving the wrong medicine, giving the right medication to the wrong child, administering the right medicine by the wrong method (route), giving the wrong dose (amount), or giving the medication at the wrong time are all medication errors. It is also a medication error if the correct dose of the medication was given twice at one time, or if the medication that the doctor ordered was not given as it was supposed to be given.

A great deal of caution and attention is necessary to avoid medication errors during administration. First, it is helpful to keep a master list of medications that are to be given in the classroom or school, the time, and the child who will receive the medication. (See Table 6-1.) Medications should be given within 15 minutes of the prescribed time.

When it is time to give a medicine, gather equipment. Remove the medicine from the locked medication storage area. Wash your hands. Prepare and administer medication for only one child at a time.

Regardless of the route, all medication should be checked three times. Double check the medication label when you take it out of the storage area. Read the name of the medication and the name

TABLE 6-1. Sample Master Medication Schedule.

ADMINISTRATION TIME	MONDAY	TUESDAY	WEDNESDAY	THURSDAY	FRIDAY	CHILD'S NAME	MEDICINE'S NAME
8:00 A.M.							
8:30							
9:00							
9:30							
10:00							
10:30							
11:00							
11:30							
12:00 P.M.							
12:30							
1:00							
1:30							
2:00							
2:30							
3:00							
3:30							
4:00							
4:30							
5:00							

of the child to be sure you have the correct bottle. After preparing the medicine (pouring it from the bottle, and so on), check the medication label again. Perform one last check before you actually give the medication to the child. Giving medication to the wrong child could have life-threatening consequences. You cannot be too careful.

Children are occasionally poisoned by accidentally ingesting medications they think are candy. In order to avoid this situation, do not give the medication in front of other children. Also, avoid referring to medication as candy.

Another basic rule of medication administration is never give a medication you did not prepare, and don't let someone else give a medication you have removed from the original container. These actions are a potential source of medication errors and can be easily avoided.

Unfortunately, medication errors do sometimes occur. If you do make an error in medication administration, call the school nurse or the child's physician immediately. Tell the nurse or physician the name of the medication and the dose the child was supposed to take, and what the child actually took. The nurse or physician will tell you the possible reactions to look for, or whether an antidote or vomiting is indicated.

Actual Administration of Medication

There are several ways (routes) by which a medication may be given in the school setting. The method is determined by the doctor's order (prescription) and considers the child's developmental age, and ability to chew and swallow. It is critical that the medication be given by the route ordered by the physician, and that it is administered correctly.

Oral (through the mouth)

Liquid Many medications given to babies and young children are liquid. Frequently, the medication container has a dropper with measurements on the side. You can use this dropper to draw up and administer the medication. The dropper is often accurate only for that type of medication, so do not use one from a different medicine. Be sure to double check that you have drawn up the correct amount. Be careful, since many droppers have markers in both cubic centimeters (ccs) and teaspoons. Be sure to use the same unit that is listed on the prescription. An even more reliable method is to use a plastic syringe with calibrations on the side to measure the correct amount of medicine. Keep an individual one for each child. An individual child's syringe may be marked with tape to indicate the correct dose.

When giving the medication with a dropper or syringe, do not direct the stream of medication directly to the back of the mouth, because you may cause the child to start choking. Rather, direct the liquid to the inside of the child's cheek. It can then be swallowed more slowly. If the child has tongue thrust, the medication may be pushed forward and out of the mouth. That medication should be collected with a spoon and readministered.

Many medications are prescribed in teaspoons. Be aware that ordinary kitchen teaspoons and tablespoons are not standardized. If you use kitchen utensils, you may be over or under-medicating the child. The standard measurement is that one prescribed teaspoon is equal to 5 milliliters (ml) or cubic centimeters (ccs) (Whaley & Wong, 1987).

Do not mix liquid medication with milk or any other fluid without the doctor's permission. There are several reasons for this guideline. First, many medications cannot be mixed with milk. The pharmacist can give information regarding specific prescriptions. Second, be sure that the child takes all the prescribed medication. If it is placed in a bottle, and the child does not drink the entire contents, you will not be sure how much of the medication was consumed. It is preferable to give the medication first, and then give other liquids or soft foods, or mix the medication in only a small amount of liquid or food. Since the medication may have a bad taste, do not mix medication with a primary food such as formula. The child may develop an aversion to the food associated with the taste of the medication.

Tablets   Children under 5 years of age cannot take tablets safely. Neither can many older children with developmental disabilities. So, tablets may need to be crushed prior to administration. However, some tablets, such as those designed for gradual release of the ingredients over many hours (time-released), cannot be crushed. Confirm with the physician or pharmacist.

To administer a tablet, take it out of the original container and put it into a cup or container. Label the cup with the name of the child and the name of the medication. Keep the original container nearby for future double-checking. Do not have other medications in the immediate area.

To crush a tablet, put it into a bowl and crush it between two spoons. If only a portion of the tablet has been prescribed, score the tablet with a knife, break the tablet into the desired size, and proceed in crushing the required amount.

After the tablet has been crushed, it can be mixed with a small amount of liquid or soft food and administered. (Check with the physician or pharmacist to be sure the tablet can be mixed with milk.)

Positioning for oral medication   Choking is a frequent problem with oral medications. To minimize choking, be sure the child is awake before attempting to administer the medication. Do not give it if the child is crying.

If the child is an infant or toddler, elevate the child's head a minimum of 15%, by using a pillow or placing the child in a sitting position. If the child is older, a sitting position should be assumed. Cooperation is often enhanced if the child is able to assist in the medication administration.

By Feeding Tube

At times, a child may receive medications by nasogastric or gastrostomy feeding tubes. (Refer to later sections of this chapter for more complete discussions on feeding tubes.)

To prevent obstruction of the feeding tube, liquid medication is preferable. If medication in a tablet must be used, crush it and mix it well with a small amount of water, formula, milk or juice before putting it in the feeding syringe (Huth & O'Brien, 1987). Remember not to crush time-released tablets or capsules.

Give the medication first, followed by the feeding. This method ensures that the medication will reach the child's stomach. Rinse the catheter with water prior to and after giving the medication to minimize clogging and to keep the medication from being mixed with the feeding or another medication (Huddleston & Ferraro, 1991). Check with the physician regarding the amount of water to use, because it may need to be considered as part of the child's total fluid intake.

Rectal (placed in the child's rectum)

Some medications must be administered by rectum. These medications are usually prescribed when the child is unable to swallow, or has been vomiting. Medications given by rectum are generally packaged in a glycerine-based suppository. To administer a suppository, obtain a latex glove and some water-based lubricating gel. Take the suppository out of the wrapper. Apply the lubricating gel to the pointed end of the suppository and to the end of the glove-covered index finger. Position the child so you can see the rectum. Hold the child with one hand to retain the desirable position. Use the covered hand to insert the suppository until you meet resistance. That is the sphincter muscle. Apply continuing gentle pressure and the suppository will slip further inside the lower intestine. Remove your finger and hold the sides of the rectum together for about 5 to 10 minutes to let the anal sphincter relax, thus avoiding expulsion of the suppository (Whaley & Wong, 1987). The presence of the suppository is not painful to the child. It will melt quickly and be absorbed by the intestine.

Topical (placed on the child's skin)

Many ointments and creams are applied to the skin. These medications may directly treat the skin itself, or may be absorbed through the skin for more general effect. To apply a topical medication, be sure the area of the skin is clean and dry. Put a small amount of topical medication on a clean cotton-tipped applicator. Do not let the tip of the tube touch your hands or the applicator itself. Use the applicator to apply the medication directly to the skin. Cover the area with a dressing, as indicated by the doctor.

Otic (placed in the child's ear)

Otic medications are applied to the ear, usually in the form of eardrops. Be sure the medications are at room temperature prior to administration. To give these medications, turn the child's head to the side and have someone hold it securely, or have the child place his head on a table, facing the side. A second person should position the child's ear by gently pulling the ear of an infant down and back, or an older child up and back. This will straighten out the ear canal and facilitate instillation of the medication. Massage the area just in front of the ear to facilitate absorption.

Ophthalmologic (placed in the child's eye)

Ophthalmologic medications are placed in the eye, usually in the form of eye drops. To administer a medication to a child's eye, have the child lie on his back, with someone else securing the child's head. If the child is able, request that the child look as far back on the ceiling as possible. Pull the lower eyelid down slightly to make a small pocket. Rest the hand holding the medicine dropper on the child's forehead or cheek, so you can move your hand in concert with any head movements. Drop the prescribed amount of medication into the pocket, taking care not to touch the end of the medication dropper or tube, or to allow the tube to touch the child's eye. Gently, let the lower eyelid return to its original position. The medication will automatically be spread across the eye. Wipe off excess medication from around the child's eye. Applying the medication into the lower lid when the child is asleep may be effective with infants.

Common Problems with Medication Administration

Problems with medication administration tend to fall into several categories.

Omission

Perhaps the most common medication problem is failure to receive the medication. Most frequently this is because the caregiver or parent forgot to give it to the child. Written schedules serve as a useful reminder.

Sometimes the medication is omitted because the child refuses to take it. Do not force the child. Attempt to determine the cause for the refusal. It may be related to oral defensiveness, or dislike of the taste, texture, or size. Sometimes, the medication may be mixed with a nonprimary food or broken into smaller pieces. If the child totally refuses to take the medication, wait 20 minutes and try again. Distraction techniques and positive reinforcement are helpful.

Overmedication

Overmedication tends to occur in two situations. The first is when the caregiver does not fully understand the potentially deadly effects of overmedication. The caregiver may erroneously assume that if the regular dose of medication did not seem to have the desired effects, then more is needed. This is not only incorrect, it could be fatal.

Overmedication also occurs if two doses are accurately given, but are given too close together. This happens if the caregiver does not remember when the last dose was given and gives a second dose by mistake. It can also happen if the child was given the medication by the parent at home, before school, and the caregiver at school gives another dose. For example, the child had an elevated temperature in the morning. The mother gave a dose of Acetaminophen at 7:00 A.M. The teacher at school noticed the child had an elevated temperature at 9:00 A.M. but did not check with the parent to see if a dose was given previously. Rather, the teacher erroneously gave a second dose in less than the prescribed interval and overdosed the child.

Overmedication can also occur if one person gives the medication at school, and another person at school is not aware that the medication was given and gives a second dose. To prevent this, only one person should be assigned to give a medication for a particular child or room each day. Medication administration should be documented in writing as soon as it has been completed.

Choking

Infants and young children, especially those with developmental delays, often have difficulty swallowing liquid medications and tablets. Preschoolers should not be given medication by tablet, since they may not be able to chew and swallow tablets safely.

To reduce the tendency for choking, position the child in an upright position, and give medication by dropper aimed at the inside cheek of the mouth. An interdisciplinary team evaluation is indicated if the child is orally defensive. The team can develop a program of relaxation and desensitization and recommendations for techniques for medication administration.

If you are giving medication to a child who has a tendency toward choking, be sure you are familiar with techniques for dealing with the situation. (Refer to Chapter 9 for a discussion of emergency measures.)

Spitting-Up

Infants and young children often spit-up liquids they have consumed. If spitting-up occurs, do not readminister the medication unless you are sure the child did not consume any of it.

Vomiting

If an infant or child vomits, do not readminister medication. There are two reasons. First, you may not be sure how much of the medication was absorbed. Secondly, vomiting is only a symptom. The underlying cause of the vomiting should be determined. If vomiting does occur, notify the parent.

Side Effects

Most medications have side effects. These are generally mild, undesirable effects that occur in addition to the therapeutic effect.

When a physician prescribes a medication, the possible side effects are weighed against the potential advantages of the medication. Then, a decision is made about the advisability of using a particular medication.

If you are to give a medication during the school day, ask the physician about possible side effects and recommended courses of action should they be needed. Document in writing when these side effects are noted. If they are severe, contact the parent and physician. In the case of severe side effects, the dose of the medication may need to be changed, or another medication prescribed.

Allergic Reactions

A child may develop a hypersensitivity to a medication and demonstrate an allergic reaction. This occurs most frequently with antibiotics. The allergic reaction may be characterized by a rash or hives, itching, vomiting and irritability, reddened skin or difficulty breathing.

If these symptoms occur, carefully observe to be sure the child continues breathing. If breathing stops, start the rescue breathing sequence of cardiopulmonary resuscitation and call the emergency medical services system (911 in most areas). If breathing is not hampered, call the parent and doctor immediately. An immediate physician evaluation is indicated.

If an allergic reaction to the medication is confirmed by the physician, never give that medication to the child again. Note the allergic reaction in red pen on the front of the child's record and on any medication logs. Send the parents a written letter regarding the adverse reactions to the medication.

Documentation of Medication Administration

Medication administration is more than giving the medicine to the child. Several important follow-up steps are indicated. After the medication has been given, assure that the medication has been returned to safe storage. Wash your hands.

Next, it is necessary to document the medication administration on the individual child's record. Record the date, the name of the medication given, the dose, the route the medication was given (oral, rectal, topically, and so on), and the child's response. Document any unusual circumstances (i.e., the medication was not given; unusual reaction from the child) and your responses (persons contacted; emergency actions). Sign your name.

This is a legal record, and may be called into court. It is imperative that all entries be written clearly, in ink. If you make an error in your documentation, do not cross it out. Instead, draw a single line through the error, write the word "error" and your initials immediately above it, and proceed to write your entry. Do not leave blank lines between written entries. Be sure to sign each entry. If your entry covers two pages, sign your name at the end of each page.

PERFORMANCE OF A HEALTH-RELATED PROCEDURE

Just as with medication administration, the performance of a health-related procedure is a potentially dangerous activity, since mistakes could have devastating consequences. Caution must be taken to assure that the caregiver has been appropriately trained and supervised in performing the procedure correctly and in identifying possible complications and/or emergency situations.

What Health-Related Procedures May be Done in the School Setting and Why Are They Done There?

There are numerous health-related procedures that may need to be done in the school setting. Most commonly, these procedures are related to clean intermittent catheterizations, feeding tubes, tracheostomies, and oxygen administration. Although every attempt should be made to have daily procedures done in the home by the parent, some procedures must be done several times a day, or when needed by the child.

Who Decides What Procedure a Child Should Receive?

The physician will decide what procedures must be done, and when they should be done. Most procedures are designed to fulfill basic body functions the child can not maintain without assistance. Even if the parent initiates the request, legally the physician must give written orders (directions) for it to be performed in the school setting in most areas of the country. However, both physician and parental permission must be obtained.

Physician Permission to Perform a Procedure

Physician written permission should be received prior to performing a procedure. This task can be accomplished by supplying the physician with a written form detailing the following: child's name, address, and birthdate; name and description of the procedure; required equipment and/or setting; reason for the procedure; possible unusual responses (including ones that should be reported to the physician); willingness to participate in training and support; the child's ability to assist or perform the procedure; the physician's name, address, phone number, signature; and the date of the order. (See Figure 6-4 for a sample physician permission form.) It is the responsibility of the person performing the procedure to consult with the physician for further clarification when the physician order is not clear, or if there are any questions regarding its execution in the school setting.

Figure 6-4.   Sample physician permission form.

PROCEDURES

This form must be completed for all health related procedures performed in the school setting. Procedures should be performed at school only when failure to receive such procedures could jeopardize the health of the child.

This form should be revised as needed after each acute illness or hospitalization. The maximum period of authorization is for one year.

Child's Name: _____ Child's Date of Birth _____

Child's Address: _____

The above child is under my medical supervision. I have prescribed the following procedure and am willing to participate in any necessary training of school personnel.

Name and Detailed Description of the Procedure: _____

Recommended Equipment and/or Setting: _____

Special Instructions or Precautions: _____

Ability of Child to Assist/Perform the Procedure: _____

Possible Adverse Responses: _____

Course of Action If Adverse Responses Should Occur (Including Identification of Adverse Responses Which Should Be Reported to the Physician):

_____

Beginning and Ending Dates for Performance in the School

_____   _____

(Beginning Date)   (Ending Date)

Physician's Name: _____ Address: _____

Phone Number: _____

Physician's Signature: _____ Date of Order _____

Parental Permission to Perform Procedures

In addition to physician authorization to perform procedures, one must also obtain parental permission. Permission forms should contain the child's name, date of birth, and address; procedure; hours the procedure should be performed; special instructions or precautions; beginning and ending dates for school performance of procedure; name and phone number of physician; authorization to perform procedure in the school; release of claim of liability for care by nonmedical personnel who have been trained in the procedure; parental agreement to let school personnel communicate freely with the physician regarding the child's care; agreement to notify the school of any changes in the procedure; parental agreement to provide equipment to the school and obtain refills of supplies as indicated; parental name, address, phone number, signature and date. (See Figure 6-5 for a sample parental permission form.)

Training Regarding Performance of Procedures

Prior to performing any procedure, the school professional should be trained by a registered nurse or the child's physician. The training should include how to perform the procedure, identification of adverse and emergency reactions and appropriate responses, recording, and actual supervision of the procedure being performed by the learner. The instructor should document in writing that you have been trained, components of the training, and that you successfully demonstrated safe and accurate performance of the procedure. These statements will provide legal verification that you were appropriately trained.

Since these comments help to transfer some legal responsibility to the instructor, the registered nurse or physician may wish to periodically re-evaluate your competency. This is to your advantage and should be encouraged. Document periodic supervision of your ability to perform the procedure safely and accurately. This will serve to document your ongoing competency to perform these activities.

Equipment Storage

It is the parent's responsibility to assure that equipment and supplies have been purchased and transported to the school. It is the responsibility of the school to provide safe storage of the equipment and supplies and safe return back to the parent.

Equipment should be stored in a secure place, so other children do not damage or alter the materials. Materials should be labeled with the child's name and not shared with other children.

It is the parent's responsibility to refill supplies as necessary. Check equipment, supplies, and medication daily to be sure there are adequate amounts. Notify parents when supplies start to get low, to allow time for refilling. Careful planning avoids unnecessary disruptions of treatment regimens.

Figure 6-5. Sample parental permission form.

PROCEDURE

This form must be completed for all procedures to be performed in the school setting. Procedures should be administered at school only when failure to receive such procedures could jeopardize the health of the child. This form should be revised as needed after each acute illness or hospitalization. The maximum period of authorization is for one year.

Child's Name: _____ Child's Date of Birth _____

Child's Address: _____

Name of Procedure: _____

Times Procedure Is To Be Performed: _____

Special Instructions or Precautions: _____

Dates for beginning and ending the performance of the procedure in the school: _____

Physician's Name: _____

Phone Number: _____

I hereby request that my child receive the above procedure while in school and away from school for official activities. I understand that this service may be performed by non-medical personnel. I grant my permission for appropriate personnel to communicate freely with my child's physician in order to manage my child's care. I understand the procedure will not be started until physician and parental permission is on file and the appropriate personnel have been trained. I understand that the law provides that there shall be no liability for civil damages as a result of the performance of this procedure where the person administering the procedure acts as an ordinarily reasonable and prudent person would under the same or similar circumstances.

I understand that I must notify the school of any changes in my child's condition or procedure. I further understand that I am responsible for ensuring the equipment safely arrives at school and for getting refills of the supplies as indicated.

_____   _____
      Parent's Signature   Date

Note: This form should be completed by parent or legal guardian.

Time Management of Procedures

If the wrong treatment is given or a treatment is given to the wrong child, it is an error. A great deal of caution and attention is necessary to avoid errors in procedure.

First, it is helpful to keep a master list of all procedures that are to be given in the classroom or school, the time, and the child who will receive the procedure. (See Table 6-2.) Procedures should be given within 20 minutes of the prescribed time.

Documentation of Performance of Procedure

Performance of a procedure is more than just completing the procedure. Several important follow-up steps are indicated. After the procedure has been completed, and the child is safe and comfortable, clean and return all equipment to a secure storage space. Wash your hands.

Next, it is necessary to document the performance of the procedure on the individual child's record. Record the date, the name of the procedure, the time, and the child's response. Document any unusual circumstances (i.e., the procedure was not completed; unusual reaction from the child) and your responses (persons contacted; emergency actions). Sign your name.

This is a legal record, and may be called into court. So, it is imperative that all entries be written clearly, in ink. If you make an error in your documentation, do not cross it out. Instead, draw a single line through the error, write the word "error" and your initials immediately above it, and proceed to write your entry. Do not leave blank lines between written entries. Be sure to sign each entry. Since your name at the end of the page, if your entry covers two pages.

This section has discussed general guidelines for performing health-related procedures in the school setting. The remainder of this chapter will discuss specific procedures.

CLEAN INTERMITTENT CATHETERIZATION

Children with spina bifida and other nervous system problems may also suffer from bladder problems. Many of these children have a condition known as neurogenic bladder. With this condition, the child is neurologically unable to control bladder emptying. The child is unable to determine if the bladder is full and in need of emptying. The bladder muscles are also dysfunctional. As a result, the bladder

TABLE 6-2. Sample Master Procedure Schedule.

ADMINISTRATION TIME	MONDAY	TUESDAY	WEDNESDAY	THURSDAY	FRIDAY	CHILD'S NAME	PROCEDURE NAME
8:00 A.M.							
8:30							
9:00							
9:30							
10:00							
10:30							
11:00							
11:30							
12:00 P.M.							
12:30							
1:00							
1:30							
2:00							
2:30							
3:00							
3:30							
4:00							
4:30							
5:00							

may become overdistended. The resultant pressure can cause backflow of urine into the kidneys and lead to kidney infection and malfunction.

Poor muscle function may also cause the bladder to empty too frequently or irregularly. As a result, urinary dribbling may occur. Due to poor nerve sensation, the child may be unaware of wetness from urinary overflow or automatic emptying. In addition to social problems and lowered self-esteem, these conditions can also lead to urinary and kidney infection and damage.

Clean intermittent catheterization (CIC) is a technique that provides regular bladder emptying. It is often prescribed by the child's physician to reduce infection and incontinence and preserve urinary tract function.

Overview

Clean intermittent catheterization involves the use of a small plastic tube (catheter) being inserted through the urinary meatus (external opening) and into the bladder. This procedure is similar to sterile urinary catheterization, except a clean rather than sterile technique is used.

Most children need to receive clean intermittent catheterization upon rising in the morning, at bedtime, and every 3 to 4 hours throughout the day to promote regular bladder emptying. (The child's physician will determine the exact time intervals most appropriate for an individual child.) Whenever possible, schedule catheterizations around significant school activities and meals, so routines will be as normalized as possible.

This procedure is not painful. Whenever possible, the child should be encouraged to assist with the procedure. This assistance promotes self-esteem and contributes to later ability to self-catheterize, thus promoting independence.

Preparation

Gather equipment for clean intermittent catheterization. Necessary equipment includes the following:

1. Catheter (size to be determined by the child's doctor)
2. Shallow pan or toilet for collecting urine
3. Soap and water
4. Unsterile latex gloves
5. Clean towels to put under the child (if indicated)
6. Cotton balls (16-20)

7. Water soluble lubricant
8. Sealable bag or other container for catheter storage
9. Plastic bag for disposal of contaminated material
10. Swab-type applicator
11. 1:10 household bleach solution for cleaning (1 part household bleach mixed in 10 parts water)

Place the equipment on a clean surface in a quiet, private location. This location should be within easy reach of the child. Explain the procedure to the child, using developmentally appropriate language. Wash your hands. Have the child handwash also, and assist, as appropriate. Put on gloves, and position the child for the procedure. This will entail removing or rearranging the child's clothing, so it does not become wet during the procedure. If the child is old enough, and can sit independently, a toilet can be used. If that position is not possible, the child may be positioned on the back on a bed or similar flat surface, with the head slightly elevated, feet flat on the bed, and knees flexed and apart.

Identify the appropriate anatomical landmarks. At this point, the procedure varies slightly for boys and girls.

Procedure: Clean Intermittent Catheterization for Boys

1. Cleanse the penis. Grasp the penis below the gland and hold it at a 45 degree angle. If the child is not circumcised, gently retract the foreskin as far as it will go without forcing it. Wash the penis with soapy cotton balls. Begin at the opening of the urethra, and using a circular motion, move outward and downward towards the base of the penis. Do this three times, using clean cotton balls each time. Rinse with clean cotton balls, using the same technique.
2. Apply a generous amount of water soluble lubricant around the urethral opening, using a swab-type applicator.
3. Apply water soluble lubricant to the catheter tip and down the catheter about 2 inches. Put the other end of the catheter into the appropriate receptacle, to collect the urine.
4. Hold the penis erect (upward and outward from the body). Grasp the sides of the penis rather than pinching the top and bottom. This position minimizes trauma.
5. With your other hand, grasp the tip of the catheter approximately 2 inches from the tip. Gently insert the catheter into the urethral opening until the urine begins to flow into the collection container. Then insert another inch.
6. Let the urine flow continue until it stops.

7. Slowly and gently, remove the catheter. If the urine begins to flow again, stop removing the tube. Allow the urine flow to continue until it stops. Then attempt to remove the tube once again. (See Figure 6-6.)

Procedure: Clean Intermittent Catheterization for Girls

1. Cleanse the genitalia with soapy cotton balls. With one hand, separate the labia, exposing the urinary opening, meatus. Place a cotton ball above the urinary opening; with a down stroke toward the rectum, cleanse the meatus. Do not clean back and forth, since bacteria from the rectal area can cause infection if it enters the meatus. Discard the cotton balls in a plastic bag. Do this three times, using clean cotton balls each time. Rinse the area using clean cotton balls and clean water. Then, use a dry cotton ball to dry the area.

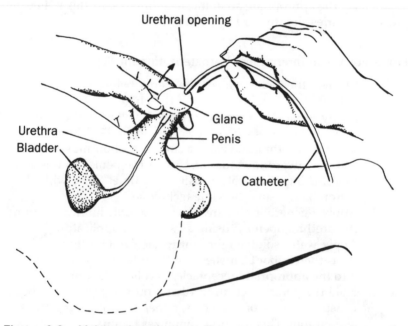

Figure 6-6. Male catheterization. The procedure used to insert the catheter through the urethra in the penis into the bladder. Reprinted from *Health care for students with disabilities: An illustrated medical guide for the classroom* by J. Carolyn Graff, R.N., M.N., p. 249, with permission of Paul H. Brookes Publishing Company, P.O. Box 10624, Baltimore, MD 21285-0624.

2. If the child is lying down, position a shallow pan between the child's thighs, for urine collection.
3. Gently, apply a water soluble lubricant in and around the urethral opening, using a swab-type applicator. Some girls may not need this lubrication.
4. Apply water soluble lubricant to the catheter tip and down the catheter about 2 inches. Put the other end of the catheter into the appropriate receptacle, to collect the urine.
5. Continue separating the labia with one hand. With the other, hold the catheter approximately 3 inches from the tip. Insert the catheter into the meatus, in a downward and backward direction, until the urine begins to flow into the collection container. Then insert another inch.
6. Let the urine flow continue until it stops.
7. Slowly and gently, remove the catheter. If the urine begins to flow again, stop removing the tube. Allow the urine flow to continue until it stops. Then attempt to remove the tube once again. (Refer to Figure 6-7.)

Followup

Following the procedure, wash the child's genitalia once again, if indicated, to remove any urine that has spilled. This helps to prevent odor. Make sure the child is dry and comfortable. Assist the child to redress, as necessary. Some children may not be able to achieve dryness, despite careful management. These children may benefit from one of several types of specially designed underpants or absorbent liners used with regular underwear.

Wash the catheter, collection container, and other equipment in soapy water. (Lather gloved hands with soap, then wash the catheter and equipment with soapy water, both inside and outside.) Rinse thoroughly. This catheter can be reused several times, if it is washed properly and stored in a plastic bag or other designated container.

Sometimes, the physician will request that all fluid the child consumes and all urine is measured. This technique is used to determine if the child is retaining fluid. If requested, measure the amount of urine, record and then discard the urine.

Cleanse the work area, and wash your hands.

Possible Problems

Resistance

You may feel slight resistance as the catheter passes through the bladder sphincters, however, gentle pressure should facilitate ad-

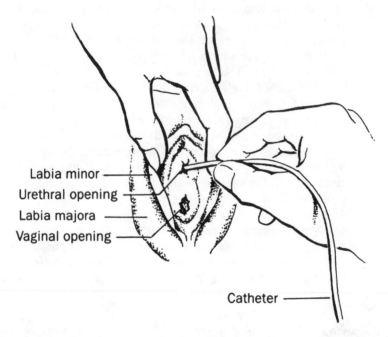

Labia minor

Urethral opening

Labia majora

Vaginal opening

Catheter

Figure 6-7. Female catheterization. The procedure used to insert the catheter through the urethra into the bladder for the female student. Reprinted from *Health care for students with disabilities: An illustrated medical guide for the classroom* by J. Carolyn Graff, R.N., M.N., p. 250, with permission of Paul H. Brookes Publishing Company, P.O. Box 10624, Baltimore, MD 21285-0624.

vancement. If it does not, change the angle of insertion slightly, or try the get the child to take in a deep breath, to relax. If strong resistance is encountered, remove the catheter and notify the child's physician, immediately.

Dropped Catheter

If the catheter is dropped or inadvertently inserted into the vagina, wash and rinse the catheter and complete the procedure (Graff, et al., 1990).

Bleeding

A small amount of bleeding may indicate the need for additional lubrication prior to catheter insertion. Blood in the urine should be reported to the physician.

Soreness, Swelling, and Discharge

Minor complications such as urethral soreness, swelling, and discharge usually indicate incorrect technique (Lozes, 1988).

Do *not* put hard pressure on the bladder, by placing your hand on the abdomen and pressuring downward, unless specifically instructed to do by the physician. This may cause internal injury.

Infection

Children who undergo catheterization are at high risk for urinary tract infection, although sometimes these infections do not have obvious symptoms. In the absence of flu or viral symptoms, notify the parents and physician if the child has a fever of 101 degrees Fahrenheit or greater.

Notify the parents and physician of the following signs of possible infection or complications: cloudy or unusual color to the urine; foul smelling urine or strong smelling urine; or excessive wetting between catheterizations.

Urinary Frequency, Urgency, or Burning

Children who need clean intermittent catheterization do not have normal neurological sensation, so they do not usually complain of urinary frequency, urgency or burning. If they do, or if unusual wetting between catheterizations is noted, report these symptoms to the physician.

Signs of an Emergency

This procedure is relatively safe and not associated with major complications (Lozes, 1988). Excessive pain or excessive bleeding should not occur. If it does, contact the emergency medical services system (911 in most areas).

Documentation

Following the completion of the procedure, record the procedure and results. If any unusual symptoms were noted, document their presence and subsequent actions.

TUBE FEEDINGS

An increasing number of children in preschool centers receive some or all of their nutrients by tube feedings rather than by mouth.

These tubes are used when a child has immature or dysfunctional oral/motor development, resulting in an inability to chew or swallow properly. They are also used if the child has a serious chronic illness that interferes with oral feedings or dysfunctional or injured areas of the upper gastrointestinal tract. Finally, feeding tubes are used if the child is too weak to eat or needs supplementary nutrition or medications.

Overview

There are generally two types of feeding tubes used in community-based settings. These types are the nasogastric tube and the gastrostomy tube.

Nasogastric tubes are used for short periods of time, to increase or improve nutritive intake, or facilitate healing by allowing food to bypass an injured area. The nasogastric tube is a small, plastic tube that is inserted through the child's nose, through the esophagus, and into the digestive track. One end of the tube remains outside the child, and the other is positioned directly into the stomach. This tubing permits liquid feedings to be delivered directly to the stomach, without direct contact with the upper gastrointestinal track itself. (Refer to Figure 6-8 for a picture of the path that the nasogastric tube takes, as well as the reference distances used to measure the length of the nasogastric tube.)

A nasogastric tube is used as a temporary measure. It can be inserted at each feeding and then removed, or it can be left in place for several days or weeks (depending on the type of tubing used).

A gastrostomy is a surgically made opening into the stomach. A gastrostomy tube is a piece of tubing used to administer food or fluids through the gastrostomy and into the stomach. Most gastrostomy tubes are used for longer periods of time, and are clamped between feedings to prevent leakage of stomach contents. They can also be used to release air or gas from the intestinal tract, if necessary. Gastrostomy tubes are more comfortable and more psychologically acceptable than nasogastric tubes. (Refer to Figure 6-9 for a picture of a gastrostomy tube.)

Selection, Preparation, and Storage of Feeding

The actual feeding formula is a liquid meal. It may be a commercial formula or a home-made blenderized mixture. The child's physician will determine the exact type of feeding a child will receive. Because the type of feeding will be chosen to meet specific medical needs, the prescribed feeding should be given with the same care used in

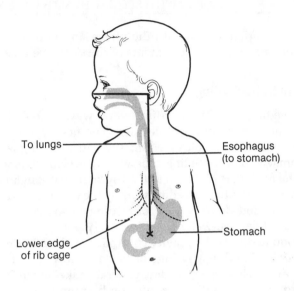

Figure 6-8. The measurement of the nasogastric tube which will pass through a nostril, down the throat and esophagus, and into the stomach. Reproduced by permission from Wong, Donna and Whaley, Lucille F.: *Clinical manual of pediatric nursing.* ed. 3, St. Louis, 1990, Mosby-Year Book, Inc.

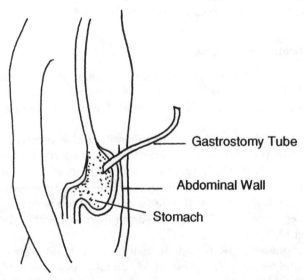

Figure 6-9. The gastrostomy tube passses through a hole in the abdominal wall and directly into the stomach.

giving a medication. Check with the physician to determine special preparation and storage requirements of the prescribed feeding.

Methods of Tube Feeding

Tube feedings can be given in several ways. The child's doctor will determine which one will be used. The first type of feeding is the bolus method. In a bolus feeding, the entire feeding is delivered to the stomach, via the feeding tube within a relatively short period of time. The feeding is placed in a 60 ml syringe (without an irrigating tip), and is pushed into the feeding tube by the plunger on the syringe. Since this method delivers a lot of feeding to the child quickly, it is not always tolerated well by children.

A second method is by gravity controlled feeding. In this method, the feeding is placed in a syringe or bag and flows into the feeding tube by gravity. This type of feeding generally takes about 30 minutes.

A third method, continuous infusion by pump, uses an infusion pump to present a regulated volume of feeding over an extended period (up to 24 hours). This type of feeding is used when a child cannot tolerate a large amount of feeding at one time. This feeding approach means the child will be connected to the feeding pump machine for prolonged periods of time. This type of feeding is not generally done in early intervention settings. Consult the child's physician if you are asked to perform this feeding.

Normalization of Feeding

Whenever possible, plan a feeding to coincide with routine mealtime activities. Since eating is a social as well as physiological activity, it is important to provide as normal a mealtime environment as possible.

Many children with feeding tubes may also receive feeding by mouth. Ask the child's physician if that is suitable for the child in your care. If it is, the physician, in consultation with an interdisciplinary feeding team, can determine the appropriate foods, consistencies, and so on. If able to consume foods orally, the child may receive feedings by mouth simultaneously with tube feedings (Graff, et al., 1990).

To promote growth and development, infants who are unable to take oral feedings should be held "en face" position while sucking a nipple. Older children can be encouraged to use developmentally age-appropriate eating utensils for oral stimulation. A child who cannot feed orally can still benefit from manipulation of task-appropriate objects.

Even though the child may not be consuming foods and fluids orally, the child's teeth and mouth should be cleansed twice daily. This will avoid unnecessary dental care and mouth infections.

Preparation

Initial preparation for a tube feeding is similar, regardless of whether a nasogastric or gastrostomy tube will be used. At that time, gather all necessary equipment:

1. Liquid gastrostomy feeding;
2. Container to measure feeding;
3. Feeding bags or 60 ml syringe with an irrigating tip;
4. Tubing;
5. Cup of water to flush out the tubing;
6. Stethoscope to check the internal position of the tube;
7. Paper or hypo-allergenic tape;
8. Clamp;
9. Pole on which to suspend the feeding bag;
10. Infusion pump, if indicated;
11. Backup suctioning equipment readily available, for use in emergency.

Place the equipment on a clean surface. Wash hands. Prepare the feeding for administration. Most feedings must be given at room temperature. Measure out only the amount to be given at the tube feeding. Place that in the feeding bag so it can begin to warm naturally. Once open, the feeding container will no longer be sterile. As with any other food, the feeding formula must be promptly used or refrigerated for future use. Label the formula with the child's name and the date, so the prescription feeding meant for one child will not be mistakenly given to another. If the formula is not used in 24 to 48 hours, discard it (Graff, et al., 1990).

Explain the procedure to the child at the appropriate developmental level. Position the child properly to facilitate safe, efficient feeding. If possible, hold the infant or child in your arms, in an upright (35-45 degree) position or place the child in a chair in a sitting position.

Procedure

At this point, the procedures for nasogastic and gastrostomy tube feedings vary somewhat.

Nasogastric Gravity Feeding

Non-nurses in schools are not generally required to actually insert the nasogastric tube. If you are required to perform this procedure, make arrangements to receive special training from the child's physician.

1. Assure that the other end of the tubing is positioned in the stomach, rather than the lung. Failure to accurately assess position can result in the feeding entering the lung with pneumonia and death as possible consequences.

   The position of the nasogastric tube can be determined in two ways.

   a. The first is to use a syringe, without a needle, connected to an inserted tube. This syringe is used to aspirate (pull out) any remaining stomach contents from the previous feeding. Fully depress the plunger on a 3 cc syringe. Attach the syringe to the exterior end of the tubing and pull on the plunger very gently. If residual stomach contents are present, the material will be pulled into the syringe. If residual stomach contents are present, note the amount by using the calibrations on the side of the syringe. Push gently on the plunger of the syringe to replace the residual contents (it contains essential fluid and electrolytes). However, subtract the amount of residual stomach contents from the next feeding, so you do not overfeed the child. If you are unable to aspirate any residual stomach contents, push the tube in gently one more inch and attempt to aspirate again. Green (bile stained) contents indicates the tube has entered the duodenum; withdraw the tube 1 to 2 inches, until stomach contents can be aspirated. Since residual stomach contents are not always available, the absence of fluid is not a positive indicator of proper placement.

   b. A second method should also be used. In this procedure, use a syringe to inject .5 cc (for neonates) or up to 5 cc (large child) of air into the nasogastric tube. Simultaneously position a stethoscope over the child's stomach (left upper quadrant of the abdomen). Listen for the crackling, swishing, or gurgling sound of the air entering the stomach. Work with your nurse or physician instructor until you are sure of what you are hearing.

      It is recommended that the caregiver responsible for tube feedings be taught and supervised in both methods prior to assuming responsibility for independent feedings. If the tubing does not seem to be in the appropriate place, do not give the feeding. Replacement of the nasogastric tubing should only be done on physician's orders, and by a specially trained professional. Otherwise, contact the parents and physician.

2. If the correct position has been confirmed, tape the tube in place. The feeding can begin.
3. Pour the formula into the syringe or feeding bag. If a feeding bag is used, pour the feeding into the bag.
4. Elevate the bag and unclamp the tubing. Allow the tubing to fill with feeding prior to connecting the tubing to the feeding tube (Zechman, 1986).
5. If a syringe is used, merely unclamp the tubing, if it has been clamped since the last feeding. Refill the syringe before it empties to prevent air from entering the stomach. Follow the physician's orders (directions) regarding type, amount and method of feeding.

Gastrostomy Gravity Tube Feeding

The gastrostomy is a surgically made hole into the stomach. One type of gastrostomy (Stamm) uses a soft, flexible tube that has been surgically inserted through the abdomen into the stomach. The tube is secured during the surgery or is held in place in the stomach by a small flange (Malecot Catheter) or a small balloon on the end of the catheter (Foley).

Another type of gastrostomy (Janeway) results in an external stoma (opening) which is flush with the abdomen. The Janeway gastrostomy requires the insertion of a straight catheter into the stoma (at a predetermined depth) at each feeding. The catheter is removed after each feeding. A dressing covers the stoma between feedings. *Note:* If you are to be responsible for inserting a gastrostomy tube, you must receive individualized training from the child's physician.

A gastrostomy feeding button has been used more commonly in recent years. This button is used when the child has received a gastrostomy through a standard procedure such as the Stamm gastrostomy. When the site has had time to heal, a gastrostomy button is inserted. The button is a flexible silicone device with a mushroom shaped dome on the internal side and two small wings on the external side (Huth & O'Brien, 1987). This button covers the external end of the tubing, flush with the child's abdomen. An attached safety plug covers the opening between feedings. An external feeding tube is needed only for the feeding itself.

The gastrostomy button simplifies care and is psychologically easier to accept. However, the child must remain fairly still during the feeding, or the tubing will become dislodged. (Refer to Figure 6-10 for a picture of a gastrostomy feeding button.)

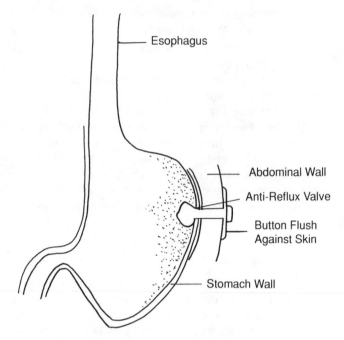

Esophagus

Abdominal Wall

Anti-Reflux Valve

Button Flush
Against Skin

Stomach Wall

Figure 6-10.   The gastrostomy button.

1. Since the gastrostomy opens directly to the stomach, it is not necessary to worry about accidental placement in the lung.
2. Use a syringe, with an irrigating tip, to aspirate (pull out) any remaining stomach contents from the previous feeding. Fully depress the plunger on the syringe, and attach it to the exterior end of the tubing. Unclamp the tubing and pull on the plunger very gently. If residual stomach contents exist, the material will be pulled into the syringe. Note the amount by using the calibrations on the side of the syringe. Push gently on the plunger of the syringe to replace the residual contents (it contains essential fluid and electrolytes). However, subtract the amount of residual stomach contents from the next feeding, so you do not overfeed the child.
3. Flush tube gastrostomies with at least 10 ccs of water (Zechman, 1986). This amount of fluid should be validated by the child's physician, because some children need to have total fluid intakes tallied daily.
4. *If the child has a gastrostomy button, modify this procedure* by using a special adaptor on the end of the feeding syringe and a

specially designed feeding tube. Open the safety plug from the button and insert the tubing into the button.

5. Clamp the gastrostomy tubing and disconnect the syringe.

6. Remove the plunger from the syringe, and reinsert the tip of the syringe into the tubing. Unclamp the tubing and allow bubbles to escape.

7. The actual feeding can then begin. Follow the physician's orders (directions) regarding type, amount and method of feeding. Since the use of a gravity controlled feeding is most commonly used in the school setting, it will be discussed here.

8. Fill the syringe or feeding bag with the prescribed amount at room temperature. If a feeding bag is used, pour the feeding into the bag. Elevate the bag and unclamp the tubing. Allow the tubing to fill with feeding prior to connecting the tubing to the feeding tube (Zechman, 1986).

9. If a syringe is used, merely unclamp the tubing, if it has been clamped since the last feeding. Refill the syringe before it empties to prevent air from entering the stomach. Allow the formula to flow by pull of gravity. (Keep the syringe at least 6 inches above the level of the stomach, or at prescribed height).

10. When approximately 5 ccs of feeding remains in the syringe, add more formula. This technique prevents air from entering the stomach.

11. Continue this procedure until the feeding is complete. The rate of the feeding can be adjusted by raising the syringe to increase the speed, and lowering it to decrease. The feeding should take 20 to 30 minutes to administer. Do not force the formula faster than prescribed. Do not allow the feeding bag or feeding syringe to become empty, as this will force unnecessary air into the child's stomach.

Followup

If a feeding bag is used, disconnect the bag from the tubing. For nasogastric, gastrostomy tube, or gastrostomy button, flush the tubing with water to rinse residual feeding from the inside of the tube. It is recommended to use 5 to 10 ccs of water for infants and 15 to 30 ccs for children (Huddleston & Ferraro, 1991). (Flush the button with water, if ordered by the physician.) Remove the syringe or feeding bag.

If the child has a gastrostomy tube, the physician may order the gastrostomy tube to be left open to air for a short period of time, to allow venting of air or gas from the intestines. This is similar to burping a baby after feeding a bottle, to remove undesirable gas buildup. Venting should be done in a private area, or as ordered by the physician. (If a button gastrostomy is in place, get instructions regarding how use of the special adaptor when venting is required.)

After the feeding, and/or venting is complete, clamp the tubing of a Staam gastrostomy and insert the cap into the end of the tubing; tape in place. (If a button gastrostomy is used, remove the adapter with the feeding syringe, and snap the safety cap into place.) If a Janeway catheter is used, remove the tubing and cover the stoma with a dressing.

Place the child in an upright position for at least 30 minutes following the feeding, to facilitate proper gastro-intestinal functioning.

Wash the equipment with warm, soapy water. To prevent the spread of infection, use the kitchen area for cleaning, rather than a bathroom sink. Store the equipment in a safe, individually marked area. Bags can be cleaned and reused for 24 hours; cleaned syringes can be reused for one week (Zechman, 1986). Wash your hands.

Possible Problems

Intolerance to Feedings

Feedings utilizing either nasogastric or gastrostomy tubes can result in intolerance to the formula. The child may show the following signs of intolerance to the formula: nausea; vomiting; diarrhea; cramping; abdominal distention (swelling). If these reactions are noted, stop or reduce the flow until the symptoms have gone. If the symptoms are still present after one hour, contact the parent and physician. Also contact them if the symptoms have occurred several times, even if they last only a short period of time. The problem may be related to allergies, intolerance of the formula, or contaminated formula.

If the symptoms have totally disappeared, the problem may be related to improper administration of the feeding. Most commonly the formula is being fed too quickly or air is entering the stomach. Be sure to use only cans of formula that have been refrigerated properly and warmed to room temperature before feeding. Investigate for possible problems with your administration technique and modify accordingly.

Rate of Flow

Intestinal signs of intolerance may occur if the feeding has entered the stomach too quickly. Gravity helps to regulate the rate of flow, so the speed of flow can be slowed down by lowering the placement bag during a feeding. The flow is further regulated by the control clamp on the feeding tube. If a feeding pump is used, the machine pumps a consistent amount of feeding in each minute. Check the indicator on the machine to be sure it is set correctly.

Temperature of the Feeding

If the feeding is too cold, abdominal cramping may occur. Be sure to check the temperature of the feeding to be sure it is at room temperature before administration. If it is too cold, stop the feeding. Bring the feeding to room temperature, then resume procedure.

Obstruction in the Tubing

As with any tube, flow of materials will be slowed down or stopped if the tubing becomes blocked or kinked. This is generally caused by inadequate flushing after feedings or medication administration.

First, check to be sure the tubing is not kinked or blocked by pressure from the child's body. If the tubing does not appear kinked, investigate the possibility that the feeding itself is too thick for the size of the tube. Using a syringe with a few ccs of water to gently flush the tubing will frequently dislodge a blockage. If medications are given in the gastrostomy tube, they may also cause blockage. Water can also be used to flush out the tubing in this situation. (Refer to the section on Medication Administration in this chapter for a discussion of giving medication by tube.)

Skin Care

Because feeding tubes and leakage of gastric contents can irritate a child's delicate skin, irritation and infection may occur. Observe for skin redness, drainage, bleeding, or foul odor in the skin area around the tube. If these symptoms are noted, notify the parent and physician.

Keep all skin around the tubing or stoma clean and dry. If a nasogastric tube is used, ask the physician about using a lubricant around the nostrils and the tube to reduce friction and potential irritation. Use non-allergic tape to secure the tubing. Use as little tape as possible. Avoid the use of lotion or powder, unless prescribed by the physician.

Do not become concerned if a small amount of bleeding is noted around the stoma. That is a normal finding.

If a gastrostomy button is used, the skin around the site should be checked daily. Obtain specific instructions regarding how to turn the button with each cleaning from the child's physician.

Blocked Gastrostomy Button

This situation may be due to thick food or fluid, or inadequate flushing of the button. Attempt to flush the button with warm water after feeding or medication administration. If you are unable to clear the blockage, contact the parents.

Leaking of Stomach Contents

Prevention through optimal positioning before and after feedings is important. This position involves placing the child on the right side, with the head of the bed elevated 30 to 40 degrees (Huddleston & Ferraro, 1991).

At times, a child's gastrostomy catheter may leak because the balloon or the flange which holds the catheter in place is not securely against the stomach wall. Pull back slightly on the tube until resistance is met. Tape it into place. If leakage continues, consult with the child's physician.

If a traditional tube is used, the leaking of stomach contents may be caused by incomplete clamping. If a gastrostomy button is used, the anti-reflux valve may not be working properly. Contact the child's physician for further instructions.

Accidental Dislodgement of Tube or Gastrostomy Button

Occasionally, a child may pull a nasogastric feeding tube or gastrostomy button out. Observe for bleeding or pain. If these do not exist, it is not a medical emergency. However, the parents and physician should be notified immediately. If the child is on continuous feedings, arrangements should be made for the tube to be reinserted promptly.

Tube gastrostomies are more permanently secured; they come out less frequently. If a tube is pulled out in the first 3 to 4 weeks after the surgery, notify the physician. It may be necessary for the physician to replace the tube. If the tube is accidentally pulled or removed after that initial postoperative period, observe for bleeding or pain. While not a life-threatening emergency, the parents and physician should be notified to assist in planning for reinsertion.

Do not throw the old tube or button away. Rather, place it in a clean cloth or container and give it to the parents for possible reinsertion. Cover the gastrostomy opening with a clean dressing and immediately notify the parent and doctor to make arrangements for tube replacement. Depending on the type of surgery, a delay of several hours may result in closure of the opening, and another surgical procedure may be needed to replace the tube.

It is not uncommon for an active child to dislodge the feeding adapter part of a gastrostomy button during feeding. If this happens, estimate the amount of feeding that was lost. Reattach the feeding adapter and continue feeding.

Signs of an Emergency

If the child chokes, coughs, gags or vomits, the feeding should be stopped immediately. The feeding should also be stopped if the child's skin color changes or if the child experiences breathing difficulty. These symptoms may indicate aspiration of the feeding into the child's lungs.

Call the nurse, if there is one available in your school. Suctioning of secretions of the mouth and back of throat may need to be conducted by a trained professional. If it is successful and the child's symptoms stop, the child should be observed and allowed to rest. Feedings can be resumed when the child is ready. If suctioning is not successful, observe for indications for cardiopulmonary resuscitation. If breathing stops, initiate resuscitation efforts and call the emergency medical services system (911 in most areas).

Documentation

Following a feeding, all equipment must be cleansed and stored in accordance with the physician's recommendations. The feeding itself should be documented by date, time, type and amount of feeding or medication, duration of feeding, child's responses, and your signature.

SUCTIONING OF THE NOSE AND MOUTH BY MACHINE

Overview

Suctioning refers to the mechanical removal of secretions that block the airway and decrease air exchange. These materials may be in the nasal passages or the mouth. If the child is not able to clear these materials independently, external suctioning is indicated.

Suctioning must be done only by someone who has been specially trained. This person is usually a physician or school nurse. However, in most states, professionals who have been especially trained by a physician, nurse or respiratory therapist are also permitted to perform this procedure. Training should include the use of the machine, insertion of the tubing, emergency use of oxygen and manual resuscitation equipment, and cardiopulmonary resuscitation. Depending on the child's age and status, it may be necessary for two trained adults to be present when performing this procedure.

Clean technique is usually ordered for suctioning of the nose and mouth. Clean technique means that clean equipment and gloves are used. Equipment does not need to be sterilized. Careful handwashing, and the use of disinfectants and warm water to clean materials is an important part of clean technique (Graff, et al., 1990). Check with the child's physician to obtain instructions for cleaning the catheter between uses. The reuse of gloves is not recommended.

The doctor may order the child to be suctioned at specific times, or as needed. *Indications for nasal suctioning* include: apparent difficulty breathing; paleness or cyanosis (bluish tinge to skin around mouth, extremities, and in nailbeds); restlessness; anxiety; noisy, rattling or gurgling breath sounds; and presence of materials that the child is unable to clear from the nasal passages. Ask the child to cough. This may expel the secretions and suctioning may be unnecessary.

Indications for oral suctioning include secretions in the mouth and back of the throat that the child is not able to cough up, or food and secretions that the child is not able to swallow or cough out. Oral suctioning is also indicated if the child has aspirated (breathed in) food, liquid or vomited material.

Since it is not always possible to pre-schedule suctioning, children in possible need of suctioning should have a suction machine, equipment, and emergency oxygen and manual resuscitation equipment (ambu bag) nearby at all times. Portable, battery powered suctioning machines should be available for use in travel to and from school. Backup suctioning equipment must be available in the event of primary machine malfunction.

Preparation

Gather equipment for suctioning. (It is recommended that the school have supplies for at least several days on hand at all times.) Necessary equipment includes:

1. Suction machine with vacuum bottle to collect secretions;
2. Suction catheter and latex glove kit (size of catheter to be determined by the child's physician);
3. Normal saline;
4. Small plastic bag that can be made airtight—for disposal of secretions;
5. Manual resuscitation equipment (ambu bag) for temporary air exchange);
6. 1:10 household bleach solution.

Place the equipment on a clean surface, in a quiet, private location. Prepare the manual resuscitation equipment (ambu bag) for easy accessibility. Wash your hands. Set suction pressure gauges as ordered by the child's physician. Check the function of the machine by turning on the machine.

Explain the procedure the child, using developmentally appropriate language. Observe for signs of respiratory difficulty and note for later documentation. Measure and note the child's pulse and respiratory rates prior to the procedure. If necessary, the child may need to be restrained by another trained adult during this procedure to prevent injury.

Measure the distance the suction tube should be inserted. This measurement is obtained by putting the tip of the catheter at the child's ear lobe and measuring the distance between that point and the tip of the child's nose (Wong & Whaley, 1990). Mark that position on the catheter, for reference during insertion. (Refer to Figure 6-11 for diagram of upper respiratory tract and Figure 6-12 for a diagram of measurement of nasogastric tube for suctioning.)

Place the child flat on the back, with head elevated (Persons, 1987). If cooperative, the child may also be sitting upright during suctioning.

Procedure

1. Open the suction and glove kit, touching only the outside.
2. Put the gloves on. (Gloves are used to prevent spread of possible infection.)
3. Attach the catheter to the suctioning tubing. Don't touch the end that will enter the child's nose and mouth.
4. If the child is capable of cooperation, ask the child to cough and take several deep breaths prior to suctioning or hyperoxygenate the child with 7 ventilations (breaths) via a manual resuscitation equipment (ambu bag); use 3 to 4 breaths for an infant.

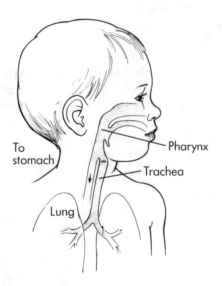

Figure 6-11. The upper respiratory tract. Reproduced by permission from Wong, Donna and Whaley, Lucille F.: *Clinical manual of pediatric nursing.* ed. 3, St. Louis, 1990, Mosby-Year Book, Inc.

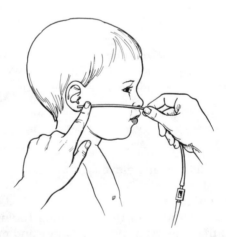

Figure 6-12. Measurement of a nasogastric tube for suctioning. Reproduced by permission from Wong, Donna and Whaley, Lucille F.: *Clinical manual of pediatric nursing.* ed. 3, St. Louis, 1990, Mosby-Year Book, Inc.

5. Turn the machine on with one hand. Using the thumb of the other hand over the catheter suction control port, draw a small amount of sterile saline through the catheter to double-check the machine function, and to clear the tubing, as necessary.

6. Use the catheter suction control port to turn the suctioning off, and introduce the catheter into one nostril at a time, or into the mouth (as indicated) to the depth you measured previously. If you are to suction both the nose and the mouth, do the nose first. If the suction tubing has no suction control port, crimp the tubing at the end nearest you, or turn the machine off to release the suction when inserting the catheter. (Refer to Figures 6-13 and Figure 6-14 for pictures of suctioning techniques.)

7. After the suction catheter has reached the desired depth, turn the suction on by removing the thumb from the catheter suction control port. Roll the catheter between the thumb and forefinger slowly as the catheter is withdrawn. Apply suction for 10 to 12 seconds at a time. **Never suction more than 5 seconds in an infant or more than 15 seconds in a child.** (If you hold your breath when your thumb is on the suction port, it will remind you of timing (Wong & Whaley,

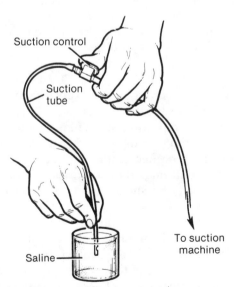

Figure 6-13. Use of the suction port. Reproduced by permission from Wong, Donna and Whaley, Lucille F.: *Clinical manual of pediatric nursing.* ed. 3, St. Louis, 1990, Mosby-Year Book, Inc.

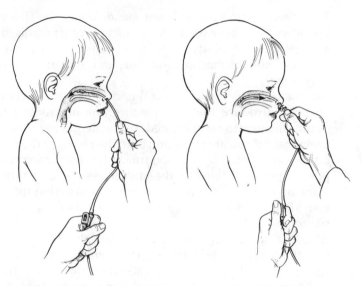

Figure 6-14. Nasal suctioning. Reproduced by permission from Wong, Donna and Whaley, Lucille F.: *Clinical manual of pediatric nursing.* ed. 3, St. Louis, 1990, Mosby-Year Book, Inc.

1990). Suction only when withdrawing the catheter. Keep the stand-by manual resuscitation equipment (ambu bag) nearby for emergency use. Suction sterile saline through the tube following each suctioning attempt, to clear the tube.

8. Repeat suctioning steps until no more secretions are seen or heard. Allow child to rest briefly between suctionings. Have the child take 7 deep breaths (30-60 seconds) between suctioning and allow coughing or expectorating, if necessary. Allow an infant to breathe for at least 30 seconds or 4 to 5 breaths before repeating suctioning. If the child is on a ventilator, interim ventilation via manual resuscitation (ambu bag) may be necessary. While the child is resting, saline can be run through the catheter periodically by putting your thumb over the suction port; this will help to keep the tubing clear.

9. After nasal suctioning is complete, the same catheter can be used to suction the mouth (Wong & Whaley, 1990). With the suction off, (thumb off the suction port), insert the suction catheter along the side of the child's mouth until it reaches the back of the throat, the cheeks, and under the tongue. Cover the suction port to apply pressure, rotate the catheter as you remove it. (**Remember never to suction for more than**

5 seconds in an infant or more than 15 seconds in a child.) Allow the child to breath between suctioning attempts. (Refer to Figure 6-15 for a diagram of oral suctioning.)

10. When suctioning is completed, hyperoxygenate child with 7 ventilations of air via manual resuscitation equipment (ambu bag), or have the child take several slow, deep breaths after the procedure has been completed.

11. Check the pulse and respiratory rate once again, and observe for unexpected variations. Observe the child's breathing— respirations should be regular and deep. The child's skin color should not be cyanotic. (Adapted from Urbano, 1989, with permission.)

Followup

Turn the machine off, and make the child comfortable, soothing as indicated. Praise the child for his or her cooperation. Return the child to usual surroundings.

Wash the catheter, collection container, and suctioning equipment with soapy water. Avoid hot water which will cook the mucus and make it difficult to remove. Rinse the inside and outside of the tube in hot running water. Shake off excess water and allow to air-dry on a paper towel. Store in a clean plastic bag (or a solution prescribed by the child's physician).

Rinse the collection container with 1:10 household bleach solution. Observe the secretions for color, odor, consistency and amount. Throw away disposable materials in the airtight plastic bag (using Universal Precautions guidelines). Cleanse work area with 1:10 household bleach solution. Wash your hands.

Possible Problems

You may feel slight resistance as the suction catheter is inserted. If you do, try to get the child to relax. Do not force the catheter.

The child may choke or gag when you insert or remove the catheter. Assure the child that you are almost finished, and proceed quickly.

If you are suctioning in the back of the throat, be very gentle. Suctioning in this area may include gagging and vomiting. If the catheter is dropped, substitute a new one. (Remember, if sterile technique is being used, a sterile replacement is needed.)

Bright red or profuse bleeding should not occur with this procedure. If profuse bleeding is noted, contact the physician immediately. A small amount of blood-tinged mucus indicates suctioning

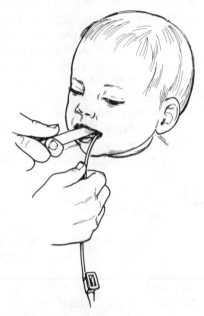

Figure 6-15. Oral suctioning. Reproduced by permission from Wong, Donna and Whaley, Lucille F.: *Clinical manual of pediatric nursing.* ed. 3, St. Louis, 1990, Mosby-Year Book, Inc.

frequency or machine pressure may need to be reduced. Be sure to use saline as a lubricant prior to insertion of the catheter.

If suctioning is ineffective, if the procedure takes too long, or if the child is not oxygenated adequately between suctioning efforts, the child may suffer increased respiratory difficulty. Adapt your procedure as indicated.

Notify the parents and physician immediately if any of the following signs of possible complications are noted:

1. Rapid pulse and respiration rate;
2. Signs of cyanosis and labored breathing which persists after suctioning;
3. Yellowish or greenish secretions;
4. Temperature elevation of 101 degrees Fahrenheit or higher;
5. Abnormally thick secretions;
6. Secretions with an unusual odor.

Note: If a child with a tracheostomy is to receive oral suctioning due to vomiting, be sure to turn the child's head to the side to avoid the entrance of the vomitus into the tracheostomy opening.

Signs of an Emergency

An emergency exists if the child is not able to breath properly or if breathing stops. Begin emergency resuscitation measures (see Chapter 9) and contact the emergency medical services team (911 in most areas).

Documentation

Following the completion of the procedure, record the procedure and results. Note color, consistency, and amount of secretions. If any unusual symptoms are noted, document their presence and subsequent actions.

SUCTIONING OF THE NOSE USING NASAL ASPIRATOR OR BULB SYRINGE

Overview

Sometimes an infant or child's nose becomes plugged with loose runny mucus, or dried, crusted mucus. In this situation, the physician may wish you to use a nasal aspirator, also known as a bulb syringe.

Preparation

Gather equipment for nasal suctioning by nasal aspirator. Necessary equipment includes:

1. Nasal Aspirator (bulb syringe);
2. Saline solution;
3. Clean eye dropper or cotton balls to insert saline into nose;
4. Tissue;
5. Gloves.

Place equipment on a clean surface. Explain the procedure to the child, using developmentally appropriate language. Observe for signs of respiratory difficulty and note for later documentation. Wash your hands. Position the child.

Procedure

1. Put on gloves.
2. Squeeze the rounded end of the bulb syringe. This is the source of suction pressure.

3. Put the tip of the bulb syringe snugly into one nostril, and release the bulb slowly. The suction pressure will suck the material from the nostril.

4. Put the pointed end of the syringe into a tissue, and squeeze. This will transfer the mucus onto the tissue.

5. Repeat steps 2 through 4 on the other nostril. (Refer to Figure 6-16 for picture of suctioning with a bulb aspirator.)

If the mucus is crusted, apply a few drops of saline into each nostril before beginning this procedure. Allow a few minutes for the saline to soften the mucus. Then continue the procedure.

Followup

Clean the bulb with tap water. Squeeze the bulb to remove water and aspirated material. Refill the bulb with water. Sterilize by boiling for 10 minutes. Empty the water from the bulb. It is then ready for reuse (Wong & Whaley, 1990).

Observe the secretions for color, consistency, and amount. Cleanse the work area. Remove your gloves and wash your hands.

Possible Problems

This is a relatively safe procedure and can be used as needed. Remember to use gentle pressure and block only one nostril at a time. Block the nostril for only short periods at a time.

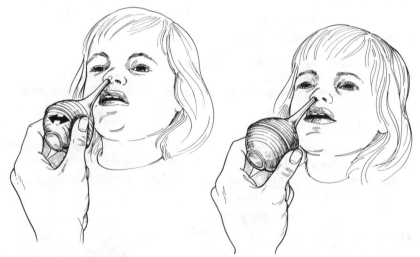

Figure 6-16. Suctioning using a bulb aspirator. Reproduced by permission from Wong, Donna and Whaley, Lucille F.: *Clinical manual of pediatric nursing.* ed. 3, St. Louis, 1990, Mosby-Year Book, Inc.

Signs of an Emergency

Emergency situations do not usually occur with this procedure.

Documentation

Following the completion of the procedure, record the procedure and the results. Note color, consistency, and amount of secretions. If any unusual symptoms are noted, document their presence and subsequent actions.

TRACHEOSTOMY MANAGEMENT

A tracheostomy is a surgically created opening (stoma) into the trachea (breathing tube). The tracheostomy is designed to improve the exchange of air in and out of the lungs, when the normal exchange through the mouth and nose has been impaired. Children with a tracheostomy may breathe normal air, or may require additional oxygen (refer to section on oxygen administration).

Tracheostomies may be done on an emergency or elective basis. They are usually performed in response to one or more of the following conditions: upper airway obstruction; laryngeal or subglottic stenosis; central nervous system trauma, and neuromuscular disease (Talabere, 1980). (See Figure 6-17 for a picture of a tracheostomy in place.)

It is necessary to keep a tracheostomy stoma open at all times. If the stoma is not kept clear and open, the child will not be able to breathe and may die. In order to keep the stoma open, a tracheostomy tube is used.

The tracheostomy tube is a hollow tube (cannula) made of metal or plastic which keeps the stoma open. The recent use of plastic and silastic tracheostomy tubes has decreased former problems with crust formation. Therefore most tracheostomy tubes used today are constructed without an inner cannula (Whaley & Wong, 1987). An additional piece, an obturator, may be used during insertion. It must be used only briefly, since its presence blocks air flow.

The tracheostomy tube is held in place by soft cotton ties placed around the child's neck. Some tracheostomy tubes also have another tube (inner cannula) which fits inside and can be easily removed for cleaning. A third piece of the tracheostomy, an obturator, is used only briefly to block the tracheostomy tube during insertion into the stoma.

Because the child's air no longer passes through the nose, procedures must be designed to replace the body's normal functions for warming, moisturizing, and humidifying the air. Adequate fluid

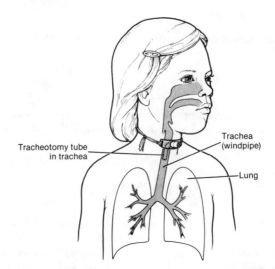

Figure 6-17. Tracheostomy tube in trachea. Reproduced by permission from Wong, Donna and Whaley, Lucille F.: *Clinical manual of pediatric nursing.* ed. 3, St. Louis, 1990, Mosby-Year Book, Inc.

intake is necessary to keep mucus liquid. A humidifier is usually kept in the child's room, to provide additional moisture. An artificial nose is also often used to provide filtering and moisture, but some children may have nothing covering the opening of the tube.

Even with a tracheostomy, many children can eat, drink, and speak normally. The child's doctor will give you specific information regarding the child's needs, if these skills are impaired. If the child is unable to speak, be sure to develop other communication techniques, so you can become aware of the child's needs.

Children with tracheostomies can usually participate in school activities, with a few extra precautions. Since the tracheostomy tube is a direct opening into the trachea, care must be taken that nothing gets into the opening. Avoid smoking, strong cleanser fumes, and aerosol sprays in the child's environment. Avoid powders and dust that may enter the airway. Take special caution that water does not enter the tracheostomy during bathing. Do not permit swimming or boating. Avoid fuzzy toys or clothing such as turtlenecks which may block the airway. Avoid sandboxes. Also, carefully observe the child to be sure no pieces of food or small toys are placed in the airway. For this reason, it is advisable to cover the tracheostomy during feeding. (Small children love to put objects into all sorts of containers, and body orifices.) A final precaution is to avoid the child's exposure to other children with infections such as cold, because respiratory infections may be especially dangerous for a child with a tracheostomy.

Initially, tracheostomy care should be provided by a registered nurse or a respiratory therapist. Later, the child's needs may become less complex and less frequent. In many situations, a child who has had a tracheostomy and is in stable medical condition may be appropriately cared for by a nonmedical care giver who has received appropriate training, with a school nurse in the building as an emergency backup (Haynie, Porter, & Palfrey, 1989.) (Refer to earlier sections for guidelines on training and appropriate permissions.) This is a team decision made by the health care team and the parent, and considers the child's medical condition, tracheostomy care needs, and responses to the school environment (Haynie, et al., 1989). The director must also consider state professional practice laws. In all cases, there should be trained personnel at the school whenever the child is present, as well as during transportation.

Although care may be assigned to a particular professional, all personnel in regular contact with a child with a tracheostomy should also have basic training in the identification of tracheostomy problems and emergency responses, and be certified in cardiopulmonary resuscitation. Equipment for routine tracheostomy care, a manual resuscitator (ambu bag), and extra tracheostomy tubes for emergency replacement should be with the child at all times (Haynie, et al., 1989).

There are several procedures that may be involved in tracheostomy management: suctioning, changing the tracheostomy tube, changing the tracheostomy ties, and skin care. **Emergency tracheostomy tube replacement, techniques to use when a tracheostomy is difficult to reinsert, and cardiopulmonary resuscitation are covered in Chapter 9, and should be reviewed prior to caring for a tracheostomy.**

SUCTIONING THE TRACHEOSTOMY

Overview

Tracheostomy suctioning refers to the mechanical removal of secretions that may block the airway. Removal is necessary to maintain an open airway, to eliminate retained or excessive secretions that may promote infection, and to promote optimal air exchange.

This procedure is usually done by a physician, school nurse, or respiratory therapist. In most states, other professionals who have been specially trained by a physician, nurse or respiratory therapist are permitted to perform this procedure. Depending on the child's age and status, it may be necessary to have two trained adults present during the procedure. Training should include the use of the machine, insertion of the tubing, emergency use of oxygen, and manual resuscitator (ambu bag), and cardiopulmonary resuscitation.

The doctor will order either sterile or clean technique to be used during tracheostomy suctioning. Sterile technique means the use of sterile equipment and gloves and great care that no equipment touches anything that is not sterile. All equipment is cleaned through the use of heat (steaming or boiling). This procedure was originally used almost extensively in the belief that sterile technique would reduce the incidence of respiratory infections.

Clean technique means that clean equipment and gloves are used. Tracheostomy care using clean technique has been found to result in fewer infections than sterile in the period following surgery (Harris & Hyman, 1984). Careful handwashing, and the use of disinfectants and warm water to clean materials is an important part of clean technique (Graff, et al., 1990). Check with the child's physician to obtain instructions for cleaning the catheter between uses. The reuse of gloves is not recommended.

Tracheostomy suctioning may be done at pre-established times, or as needed. Indications of impaired respiratory function and need of suctioning include: gurgling or bubbling of mucus heard at the opening of the trachea; coughing; increased respiratory rate or apparent trouble breathing; cyanosis (bluish tinge to skin around mouth, extremities, and in nailbeds); restlessness; anxiety.

Because it is not always possible to pre-schedule suctioning, any child with a tracheostomy should have a suction machine, equipment and emergency oxygen and manual resuscitator (ambu bag) nearby at all times. Portable, battery powered suctioning machines should be available for use in travel to and from school. Use only one machine for each child to prevent the spread of infection. Backup suctioning equipment must be available in the event of primary machine malfunction.

Preparation

Tracheostomy suctioning should be done before meals (Kennedy, Johnson, & Sturdevant, 1982; Ruben, et al., 1982). This decreases the possibility of gastro-intestinal upset. Suctioning should also be done before and after sleeping.

Gather equipment for tracheostomy suctioning. (It is recommended that the school have supplies for at least several days on hand at all times.) Necessary equipment includes:

1. Suction machine (with universal adapter, if needed), connecting tubing, and a vacuum bottle to collect secretions;

2. Sterile, nondurable catheter and latex glove kit (size of catheter to be determined by the child's physician); (clean catheter and gloves can be used if the physician orders clean technique);
3. Sterile gauze squares for use as a dressing, if ordered by the physician; (clean gauze squares if clean technique is ordered);
4. Sterile normal saline;
5. Small plastic bag that can be made airtight for disposal of secretions;
6. Oxygen source, if ordered by the child's physician;
7. Manual resuscitator (ambu bag) with tracheostomy adapter;
8. 1:10 household bleach solution.

Place the equipment on a clean surface, in a quiet, private location. Prepare the oxygen source and manual resuscitator (ambu bag) for easy accessibility. Wash hands.

Set suction pressure gauges as ordered by the child's physician. Suction pressures should not be over 100 mm Hg (millimeters of mercury) for infants or over 120 mm Hg for children (Wong & Whaley, 1990).

Plug the portable self-contained oxygen unit (if ordered) into a grounded outlet, and check the function of the machine by turning on the machine.

Go to the child. Explain the procedure to the child, using developmentally appropriate language. Observe for signs of respiratory difficulty and note for later documentation. Measure and note the child's pulse and respiratory rates prior to the procedure. If necessary, the child may need to be restrained by another trained adult during this procedure to prevent injury.

Place the child flat on the back, with head elevated (Persons, 1987). (Refer to Figure 6-18 for pictures of tracheostomy suctioning.)

Procedure

1. Open the catheter and glove kit. Put gloves on. If sterile technique is being used, put the sterile glove on one hand by removing the glove from the sterile package, holding the inside of the glove cuff and pulling the glove on with the other hand. Only sterile surfaces can touch other sterile surfaces. Use the nongloved hand to use nonsterile equipment.
2. Attach sterile (or clean) catheter to suctioning tubing. Don't touch the catheter end that will enter the tracheostomy.

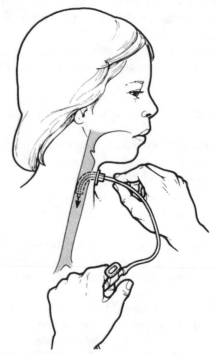

Figure 6-18. Tracheostomy suctioning. Reproduced by permission from Wong, Donna and Whaley, Lucille F.: *Clinical manual of pediatric nursing.* ed. 3, St. Louis, 1990, Mosby-Year Book, Inc.

3. If the child is capable of cooperation, ask the child to cough and take several deep breaths prior to suctioning. If not, hyperoxygenate the child with 7 ventilations (breath) via manual resuscitator (ambu bag); use 3 to 4 for an infant;

4. Turn machine on with one hand. Using the thumb of the other hand over the catheter suction control port, draw a small amount of sterile normal saline through the catheter to double-check machine function, and lubricate the tubing.

5. With dominant hand, instill sterile normal saline in the tracheostomy to liquify secretions and facilitate removal. (Amount is dependent on physician orders.) Amounts of saline should not exceed .5 ccs for infants, 1 to 2 ccs for toddlers, and 3 ccs for children (Wong & Whaley, 1990).

6. Use the catheter suction control port to turn the suctioning off, and introduce the catheter into the tracheostomy to the depth recommended by the child's physician. Usually this

is 2 to 3 inches for an infant or small child (Wong & Whaley, 1990).

If the suction tubing has no suction control port, crimp the tubing at the end nearest you, or turn the machine off to release the suction when inserting the catheter.

7. After the suction catheter has reached the desired depth, turn the suction on, by removing the thumb from the catheter suction control port. Roll the catheter between the thumb and forefinger slowly as catheter is withdrawn. Apply suction for 10 to 12 seconds at a time. **Never suction more than 5 seconds in an infant or more than 15 seconds in a child.** (If you hold your breath when your thumb is on the suction port, it will remind you of timing (Wong & Whaley, 1990.) Suction only when withdrawing catheter. Keep stand-by oxygen or manual resuscitator (ambu bag) nearby for emergency use.

8. Allow the child to rest briefly between suctionings. Have the child take 7 deep breaths (30 to 60 seconds) between suctioning and allow coughing or expectorating, if necessary. Allow an infant to breathe for at least 30 seconds or 4 to 5 breaths before repeating suctioning. If the child is on a ventilator, interim ventilation via manual resuscitator (ambu bag) may be necessary. While the child is resting, saline can be run through the catheter periodically by putting your thumb over the suction port; this step will help to keep the tubing clear.

9. Repeat steps 6, 7, and 8 several times until no more secretions are seen or heard.

10. Hyperoxygenate the child with 7 ventilations of air via manual resuscitator (ambu bag), or have the child take several slow, deep breaths after the procedure has been completed.

11. Check the pulse and respiratory rate once again, and observe for unexpected variations. Observe the child's breathing—respirations should be regular and deep. The child's skin color should not be cyanotic (bluish).

Followup

Turn the machine off, and make the child comfortable, soothing as indicated. Praise the child for cooperating. Return the child to usual surroundings.

Wash the catheter, collection container, and suctioning equipment with soapy water. Avoid hot water which will cook the mucus and make it difficult to remove. Rinse the inside and outside of the tube in hot running water. Shake off excess water and allow to air-dry on a paper towel. Store in a clean plastic bag, or a solution recommended by the child's physician.

Rinse the collection container with 1:10 household bleach solution. Observe the secretions for color, odor, consistency and amount. Throw away disposable materials in the airtight plastic bag (using Universal Precautions guidelines). Cleanse work area with 1:10 household bleach solution. Wash your hands.

Possible Problems

The saline and suctioning procedure may make the child cough. This response is normal.

You may feel slight resistance as the suction catheter is inserted. If you do, try to get the child to relax. Do not force the catheter.

If using sterile technique and the catheter is dropped or inadvertently touches anything except the inside of the tracheostomy tube, it must be discarded. A new sterile catheter must be used. If using clean technique, a new clean catheter must be substituted.

Bright red or profuse bleeding should not occur with this procedure. If it is noted, notify the parents and the physician immediately. A smaller amount of blood tinged mucus indicates suctioning frequency or machine pressure may need to be reduced.

If suctioning is ineffective, if the procedure takes too long, or if the child is not oxygenated adequately between suctioning efforts, the child may suffer increased respiratory difficulty. Adapt your procedure as indicated.

Notify the parents and physician immediately if any of the following signs of possible complications persist after suctioning:

1. Rapid pulse and respiration rate;
2. Signs of irritability, cyanosis and labored breathing which persists following suctioning;
3. Yellowish or greenish secretions;
4. Temperature elevation of 101 degrees or higher;
5. Abnormally thick secretions;
6. Secretions with an unusual odor;
7. Bright red blood coming from the tracheostomy;
8. Signs of illness, such as fever and vomiting.

Signs of an Emergency

An emergency exists if the airway becomes blocked. The addition of 1 cc of sterile water into the tracheostomy tube, and immediate suctioning may help clear the airway. If the child stops breathing, or shows signs of respiratory distress, or the tracheostomy tube is accidentally pulled out or falls out, perform emergency sterile tracheostomy tube replacement. (Refer to Chapter 9.) If the tube is accidentally pulled out, and no sterile backup is available, reinsert the old tube (Ruben, et al., 1982) and notify the physician. If breathing does not improve after the new tube has been inserted, begin mouth to tracheostomy or bag to tracheostomy ventilation and contact the local emergency medical services system (911 in most areas).

Documentation

Following the completion of the procedure, record the procedure and results. Note color, consistency, and amount of secretions. If any unusual symptoms are noted, document their presence and subsequent actions.

Note: This section describes only suctioning by machine. Tracheostomy suctioning by bulb syringe is used only when secretions have been coughed to the top of the tracheostomy. Suctioning by bulb syringe is not a substitute for deep suctioning. Do not insert a bulb syringe into the tracheostomy.

USING A MANUAL RESUSCITATOR

Overview

A manual resuscitator (ambu bag) may be used to provide additional oxygen to a child during suctioning procedures or during emergency situations.

Preparation

A manual resuscitator (ambu bag) should be available for possible use during all suctioning procedures. In addition, it should be available for possible emergencies if an electrical oxygen source is not available. Wash hands and gather equipment. Necessary equipment includes:

1. Manual resuscitator;
2. Adaptor for a tracheostomy, if the child has a tracheostomy;
3. Appropriate sized mask, if the child does not have a tracheostomy.

Place the equipment on a clean surface, in a quiet, private location. Check that the resuscitator is functioning properly. (Squeeze the bag; you should feel slight resistance.)

Explain the procedure to the child, using developmentally appropriate language. Observe for signs of respiratory difficulty and note for later documentation. Position the child. Attach resuscitator to tracheostomy tube, using the tracheostomy tube adaptor. (Refer to Figure 6-19 for a diagram of a manual resuscitator in use with a tracheostomy.)

Procedure

If the child is able to breathe, coordinate breaths from the manual resuscitator. This is done by squeezing the resuscitator bag as the child's chest begins to rise.

If the child is unable to breathe, squeeze the bag rhythmically to deliver the prescribed number of respirations per minute. If no amount is prescribed, give 20 to 24 breaths per minute for infants and 16 to 20 for children (Haynie, et al., 1989). Continue until the child has been oxygenated according to procedure.

Followup

Make sure the child is comfortable and breathing easily. Cleanse the equipment. Wash your hands.

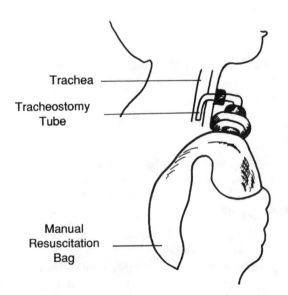

Figure 6-19. A manual resuscitator in use with a tracheostomy.

Possible Problems

If the child looks anxious or distressed, be sure you are coordinating your efforts with the child's breathing attempts.

Signs of an Emergency

If the child is unable to breathe independently, it is an emergency situation. Continue manual resuscitation and call for emergency medical assistance (911 in most areas). Continue manual resuscitation until the emergency response system team arrives and assumes responsibility.

Documentation

Document procedure, observations, actions, and the child's responses.

CHANGING THE TRACHEOSTOMY TUBE

Overview

Tracheostomy tubes should be changed regularly so the tube can be cleaned thoroughly. This procedure helps to prevent airway obstruction caused by accumulated secretions, as well as reduce subsequent infection. The child's doctor will provide guidelines for the individual child, based on the amount and type of secretions the child produces. Whenever possible, the tracheostomy tube should be changed by the parent at home. If routine tracheostomy tube changes must be done at school, they are usually done by a physician, nurse, or respiratory therapist. In most states, other professionals who have been specially trained by a physician, nurse or respiratory therapist are permitted to perform this procedure. Remember, all professionals working with a chid with a tracheostomy tube should be competent in performing emergency tracheostomy tube replacement. When changing the tracheostomy tube of a preschool-age child, it may be necessary to have two trained adults present.

The doctor will tell you whether a clean or sterile technique is to be used for a particular child. Sterile technique means the use of sterile equipment and gloves and great care that no equipment touches anything that is not sterile. All equipment is cleaned through the use of heat (steaming or boiling). This procedure was originally used almost extensively in the belief that sterile technique would reduce the incidence of respiratory infections.

Clean technique means that clean equipment and gloves are used. Tracheostomy care using clean technique has been found to result in fewer infections than sterile in the period following surgery (Harris & Hyman, 1984). Careful handwashing and the use of disinfectants and warm water to clean materials is an important part of clean technique (Graff, et al., 1990). Check with the child's physician to obtain instructions for cleaning the catheter between uses. The reuse of gloves is not recommended.

Preparation

Tracheostomy tubes should be changed 2 to 3 hours after meals, to avoid the possibility of vomiting (Wong & Whaley, 1990). Choose a time and location where you will not be interrupted. If the child is young or frightened, you may need someone to assist in restraining the child, to prevent injury.

Gather equipment for tracheostomy tube change. Necessary equipment for a routine tracheostomy tube change includes:

1. Sterile (or clean) tracheostomy tube with tracheostomy ties attached; (The child's physician will tell you whether the tube should be sterile or clean, the size and type of tube, with clean tracheostomy attached prior to tracheostomy tube change.)
2. Obturator, if indicated;
3. An extra tracheostomy tube, one size smaller, for emergency use;
4. Bandage scissors;
5. Sterile (clean) gauze squares, for use as a dressing, if ordered by the child's physician;
6. Suction unit with vacuum bottle, and suction catheter (size appropriate for the child);
7. Manual resuscitator (ambu bag) with adapter;
8. Oxygen source, if ordered by the child's physician;
9. Sterile (clean) gloves;
10. Sterile saline;
11. Hot soapy water;
12. Pipe cleaners;
13. Blanket roll;
14. Mummy wrap, if needed to restrain the child;
15. Plastic bag for disposal of contaminated items;
16. 1:10 household bleach solution.

Place the equipment on a clean surface, in a quiet, private location. Wash your hands. Prepare tracheostomy ties and place on new tracheostomy tube. Have materials for emergency tube, suctioning, and oxygen administration available, in case of emergency.

Go to the child. Explain the procedure to the child, using developmentally appropriate language. Observe for signs of respiratory difficulty and note for later documentation. Measure and note the child's pulse and respiratory rates prior to the procedure. (Refer to Figure 6-20 for a picture of a tracheostomy tube change.)

Position the child with a small blanket roll under the child's shoulders to allow the neck to bend back slightly and expose the tracheostomy stoma. (Use caution to avoid hyperextension of the neck in an infant or very young child.) Restrain the child as necessary.

Procedure

1. Suction the old tracheostomy until clear, if necessary.
2. Have one person hold the tracheostomy tube in place while the other carefully cuts the old tracheostomy ties with the rounded bandage scissors.
3. Have the second person apply a small amount of sterile saline to the far end of the new tube, to moisten it for insertion. Shake off the excess saline.
4. The first person holds the child's head in midline, and removes the old tracheostomy tube.
5. The second person inserts the new tracheostomy tube into the stoma (opening), and removes the obturator, if present. (Some tracheostomy tubes do not have obturator guides.)
6. While the second person holds the new tracheostomy tube securely in place, secure the tracheostomy ties at the side or back of the neck. (You should be able to place one finger under the secured ties.)
7. Feel for air coming out of the tracheostomy.
8. Provide 3 to 5 breaths by manual resuscitator, if needed.
9. Suction if needed.
10. If instructed by the physician, secure a clean dry adressing around the tracheostomy to keep it clean.

Followup

Remove the neck roll. Hold and comfort the child. Praise the child. Observe for unexpected variations in pulse and respiration. Respirations should be regular and deep. The child's skin should not be cyanotic (bluish). When the child's condition is stable, return the child to usual surroundings.

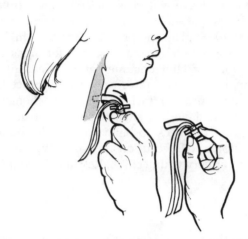

Figure 6-20.   Changing a tracheostomy tube. Reproduced by permission from Wong, Donna and Whaley, Lucille F.: *Clinical manual of pediatric nursing.* ed. 3, St. Louis, 1990, Mosby-Year Book, Inc.

Wash the tracheostomy tube and other equipment in soapy water. Avoid hot water which will cook the mucus and make it difficult to remove. Rinse the inside and outside of the tube in hot soapy water, using pipe cleaners. Rinse in hot, running water. Rinse inside and out with sterile saline (Wong & Whaley, 1990). Place inside a paper towel to dry. When drying is complete, store in a sealed, clean plastic bag. If sterile procedure is being used, sterilize equipment prior to the next use.

Rinse the collection container with 1:10 household bleach solution. Observe the secretions for color, odor, consistency, and amount. Throw away disposable materials in the airtight plastic bag (using Universal Precautions guidelines). Cleanse work area with 1:10 household bleach solution. Remove gloves and wash your hands.

Possible Problems

Coughing and/or gagging commonly occurs as the old tracheostomy tube is being removed. Assure the child that you are almost finished, and attempt to comfort him or her.

If using sterile technique and the tracheostomy tube is dropped or inadvertently touches something which is not sterile, a sterile backup tube should be used.

If you experience difficulty in inserting the new tracheostomy tube, reposition the child's head so it is tipped slightly back and spread the stoma gently. Inset the tube as the child inhales. If still unable to insert, use the smaller size tracheostomy tube. If problems still persist, and the smaller tube cannot be inserted, insert a suction catheter into the stoma to maintain an open airway. Once the child relaxes, reattempt tracheostomy tube insertion.

Notify the parents and physician immediately if any of the following signs of possible complications are noted:

1. Rapid pulse and respiration rate;
2. Signs of irritability, cyanosis, and labored breathing which persists after suctioning;
3. Yellowish or greenish secretions;
4. Temperature elevation of 101 degrees Fahrenheit or higher;
5. Abnormally thick secretions;
6. Secretions with an unusual odor;
7. Bright red blood coming from the tracheostomy.

Signs of an Emergency

An emergency exists if the airway becomes blocked or excessive bleeding occurs. If blockage occurs as a result of difficulty inserting the new tube, follow the steps indicated under Possible Problems. If they are not effective, contact the emergency medical services (911 or equivalent) and begin cardiopulmonary resuscitation. Remember to cover the child's nose and mouth, and perform emergency resuscitation through the tracheostomy stoma.

If the child stops breathing, or show signs of respiratory distress, or the tracheostomy tube is accidentally pulled out or falls out, perform emergency sterile tracheostomy tube replacement. (Refer to Chapter 9.) If no backup tube is available, reinsert the old tube and notify the physician immediately.

Documentation

Following the completion of the procedure, record the procedure and results. Note color, consistency and amount of secretions. If any unusual symptoms are noted, document their presence and subsequent actions.

CHANGING THE TRACHEOSTOMY TIES

Overview

It is necessary to change tracheostomy ties when they are soiled or the tube is changed. Usually this means ties are changed at least daily, to avoid skin irritation.

Preparation

Tracheostomy ties should be placed on tracheostomy tubes prior to tube change. They may also need to be changed on a tracheostomy tube that has been inserted into a child. (The latter procedure is described here. It incorporates critical elements for changing tracheostomy ties prior to tube change.)

Gather the following equipment:

1. Twill tape or bias tape;
2. Bandage scissors;
3. Hemostat;
4. Obturator;
5. Mummy restraint, if needed for an infant or small child;
6. Extra tracheostomy tube, suction equipment and catheter on hand, in case of emergency;
7. Gloves (sterile if sterile technique is used for this child's tracheostomy).

Place the equipment on a clean surface, in a quiet, private location. Two trained adults should be available for this procedure. Wash hands. The person who will hold the tracheostomy tube in place should put on gloves.

Go to the child. Explain the procedure to the child, using developmentally appropriate language. If necessary, the child may need to be restrained by another trained adult during this procedure, to prevent injury. Place the child with the head slightly raised.

Procedure

1. The person with the gloves should hold the tracheostomy tube in place at the outer edges (flanges). Avoid occluding the hole of the tracheostomy tube.
2. The second person moves the existing ties out of the way (but does not cut them yet). The new ties are threaded through the hole in the tube flange and secured. The hemostat can be used to help in the threading. Repeat for the other side.
3. While the tracheostomy tube is held securely in place, have the child flex the head forward. Tie the ends of the tape in the back of the neck, or to the side. The ties should be snug enough for one finger to fit under the ties.
4. Remove the old ties.

Followup

Sooth and praise the child. Observe the child to assure that breathing is normal. Then return the child to usual surroundings. Dispose of old materials. Clean other equipment and store.

Possible Problems

Secure the tracheostomy tube in place throughout the procedure to assure it is not dislodged. If it is dislodged, perform emergency tracheostomy tube replacement (see Chapter 9).

Avoid tying the ties too tightly. Tight ties contribute to difficulties in circulation and breathing and skin breakdown. If the ties are too loose, the tracheostomy tube may become dislodged.

Signs of an Emergency

If the airway is occluded, the child will not be able to breathe. Contact the emergency medical services and institute cardiopulmonary resuscitation.

If the tracheostomy tube becomes dislodged, perform emergency tracheostomy tube replacement.

Documentation

Following the completion of the procedure, record the procedure and results. If any unusual events occurs, document their occurrence and subsequent actions.

TRACHEOSTOMY SKIN CARE

Overview

The presence of humidified air around a tracheostomy and the possible existence of secretions from the tracheostomy predispose the skin surrounding the stoma to irritation. Skin care should be conducted routinely to assure optimal skin integrity.

Preparation

Routine skin preparation should be included as part of tracheostomy suctioning and tube changes. Equipment includes applicators, 50% hydrogen peroxide/water solution (or equivalent ordered by the physician), and clean or sterile gauze squares (if dressings are ordered by the child's physician).

Procedure

1. Observe the condition of the skin during other routine tracheostomy care. Observe for redness, swelling, cuts and bruises, and discharge. Note any of these observations for later documentation.
2. Clean the area surround the stoma with hydrogen peroxide and water solution. Remove dried or crusted materials.
3. Dry with gauze squares.
4. Apply medications and other topical materials only as prescribed by the child's physician.

Followup

Dispose of contaminated materials, using universal precautions for infection control.

Possible Problems

Notify the parents and physician if redness, swelling, cuts and bruises, and discharge are noted.

Avoid touching a sterile tracheostomy tube with any nonsterile materials.

Signs of an Emergency

If the tracheostomy opening is blocked, the child will not be able to breath. Immediately remove an obstruction. If unsuccessful, contact the emergency medical services system (911 or equivalent) and begin cardiopulmonary resuscitation.

Documentation

Record the procedure, observations, untoward responses, and actions taken.

OXYGEN ADMINISTRATION

Overview

Children suffering from prematurity, or pulmonary and cardiac conditions may need supplemental oxygen. These children may or may not have a tracheostomy.

The physician, in collaboration with other members of the team, will determine the child's need for oxygen and the best way to administer the oxygen. A respiratory therapist from an oxygen company is usually the person responsible for setting up and monitoring oxygen equipment. The respiratory therapist is also responsible for correcting equipment difficulties and coordinating oxygen regimes with the physician. When choosing an oxygen equipment company, it is advisable to choose one that provides 24-hour emergency service by a respiratory therapist.

In most areas, a respiratory therapist or registered nurse is assigned to supervise children on oxygen in school settings. Since the technology for nonhospital oxygen administration is changing rapidly, a complete discussion of equipment is beyond the scope of this chapter. All professionals working with children receiving oxygen should, however, understand some basic concepts of oxygen administration. Further instruction regarding the details of specific equipment usage should be provided through the child's physician and respiratory therapist.

Although the actual administration of oxygen will probably fall to the respiratory therapist and/or nurse, other members of the team share related responsibilities. First, the environment should be modified to meet oxygen administration needs. This will include making space for oxygen equipment, providing electrical sources and emergency backup generators, and removing heat sources that may cause a fire. (This includes gas for cooking and birthday candles.)

Remove any electrical devices and spark-producing mechanical toys from the room. Avoid the use of wool, silk, rayon, nylon and other fabrics prone to producing static electricity. Avoid the use of household cleaners, hairspray, and acetone (such as nail polish remover) in the room with oxygen. Also avoid the use of oil-based lotion on the caregivers hands, or the child's face.

The oxygen container should be placed on a secure holder, to avoid accidental falls. Signs should be posted prohibiting cigarette and pipe smoking. The oxygen source should also be labeled as "oxygen for medical purposes." Also post the name of the home oxygen supply company contact in an obvious place. Extra oxygen and equipment should always be kept near the child.

If the child on supplemental oxygen is transported by the school, similar precautions regarding environmental modification, training, and posting should be instituted. A two-way communication should be in effective at all times, so the bus driver can receive emergency assistance, if needed.

All professionals working with a child receiving oxygen should become familiar with the specific equipment used, accident prevention, emergency procedures, and problem-solving techniques. In addition, team members should be certified in pediatric CPR.

Professionals should be taught to constantly observe for signs such as labored breathing, cyanosis (bluish tinge to the skin, lips, or nailbeds), and increased respiratory rates that may indicate inadequate oxygenation. Difficulty eating and behavioral changes may also indicate the need for more oxygen. These symptoms should be reported to the respiratory therapist or nurse, family, and physician.

The team should also consult the physician regarding the need for adaptations in feeding, communication, exercise, and positioning. Respiratory infections are potentially deadly for a child with impaired respiratory status, so meticulous infection precautions are critical.

Oxygen Sources

Oxygen may be provided from several sources: oxygen concentrator, liquid oxygen, or cylinder oxygen. Oxygen concentrators are relatively large tanks that convert oxygen in the normal room air into a concentrated source of oxygen. These concentrators are bulky and take a lot of space. They are also dependent on electricity, so backup oxygen containers must be present for possible use in an electricity blackout. Concentrators generally are not portable and are not compatible with all types of oxygen masks.

Liquid oxygen is appropriate for small oxygen flow or to refill portable units. Cylinder oxygen refers to small, portable oxygen tanks that can be used for outings and emergency backup. The amount of oxygen available in liquid and cylinder oxygen tanks is indicated by a regulator (pressure valve) located on the tank.

Oxygen Humidification

Excessive drying of respiratory airways predisposes a child to subsequent respiratory infection. To avoid this situation, it is necessary to provide additional humidification to supplemental oxygen. A variety of devices such as nebulizers that provide a visual mist, a tracheostomy collar, or "artificial noses" are used to assure adequate humidification. If the child has thicker secretions than usual, contact the physician. Additional humidification may be needed.

Oxygen Delivery Systems

It is necessary to delivery the oxygen from the oxygen source to the child. Oxygen sources contain some type of meter or gauge that indicates how much oxygen is left in the tank, as well as a dial indicating the flow of oxygen. This amount is prescribed by the physician and should never be decreased.

The oxygen is delivered through the regulator, into a humidification device, and through clear plastic tubing to the child. The actual delivery of oxygen to the child is most commonly through devices such as: mask; nasal cannula; and ventilators.

Preparation/Procedure: Oxygenation by Mask

The oxygen mask fits over the mouth and nose, and is connected via tubing to an oxygen source, and possibly to a humidification source. The mask itself is similar in appearance to those available on airplanes. (Refer to Figure 6-21 for a diagram of an oxygen mask.)

An oxygen mask can be used for mouth or nose breathing, therefore it is useful if nasal passages are blocked. Oxygen masks come in infant, child, and adult sizes, so it is important to be sure the correct size is being used. An oxygen mask provides a wider range of oxygen concentration than is available through a nasal cannula.

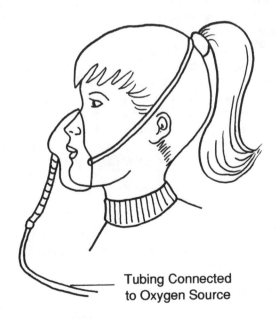

Tubing Connected
to Oxygen Source

Figure 6-21.   Oxygen mask.

In preparation for administering oxygen through a mask, gather and assemble equipment; wash your hands. Next, set the oxygen flow on the machine and the oxygen concentration on the mask valve (if present) to the levels prescribed by the child's physician. Put the mask to your face to assure air flow.

Explain the procedure to the child, using appropriate development terminology. Observe for signs of respiratory difficulty and note for later documentation. Measure and note the child's pulse and respiratory prior to the procedure.

Place the mask over the child's nose and mouth. Secure with the attached elastic band over the child's head. Assure the child is breathing normally.

Preparation/Procedure: Oxygenation by Nasal Cannula

The nasal cannula looks like a piece of tubing with two small prongs (one for each nostril). The nasal cannula is used when the child's nasal passages are clean and intact. It delivers low to moderate concentrations of oxygen. A nasal cannula will not interfere with eating, coughing, or talking. It is also connected via tubing to the oxygen and humidity sources. (Refer to Figure 6-22 for diagram of a nasal cannula.)

To administer oxygen through a nasal cannula, gather and assemble equipment, and wash your hands. Set the oxygen flow on the machine to the level prescribed by the child's physician. Put the nasal cannula to your face to assure air flow.

Explain the procedure to the child, using appropriate development terminology. Observe for signs of respiratory difficulty and note for later documentation. Measure and note the child's pulse and respiratory prior to the procedure.

Insert the two prongs of the nasal cannula into the child's nose. Make sure one prong is in each nostril. Loop the tubing over each ear and then under the child's chin. Secure by sliding the clasp under the skin. Be careful it is not too tight and that it does not rub the skin. Assure the child is breathing normally.

Followup

Make sure all equipment is functioning properly and all tubes are unkinked. Praise the child for his or her cooperation.

Clean the equipment as indicated.

Possible Problems

Oxygen administered to an infant or child well enough to leave the hospital will not cause blindness or eye damage.

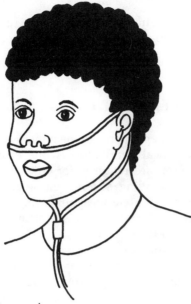

Figure 6-22.   Nasal cannula.

If the equipment does not work, check all connections and be sure the equipment is connected to the electrical source.

Skin redness, dryness or bleeding is usually related to mechanical irritation from the equipment or excessive dryness of the oxygen itself. Contact the child's physician for future course of action.

Signs of an Emergency

If the oxygen cannula or mask is removed accidentally, the child will not stop breathing. This is not an immediate emergency, but efforts should be made to resume the flow of oxygen as soon as possible.

If the child shows evidence of respiratory distress (labored breathing, cyanosis, rapid pulse and respirations, anxiety or agitation), double check equipment, oxygen flow, and position of equipment on the child's face. Be sure that tubing is not kinked and that oxygen flow from the equipment is not blocked.

If the equipment fails, institute manual respirator with a manual resuscitator (ambu bag). Refer to that section of this chapter.

If the child continues to show respiratory distress despite appropriate oxygen levels, stops breathing or becomes unconscious, institute cardiopulmonary resuscitation, as indicated. (Refer to Chapter 9.)

Documentation

Following the completion of this procedure, record the procedure and results. If any unusual symptoms are noted, document their presence and subsequent actions.

MECHANICAL VENTILATION

Some children are dependent on machinery for support of basic life functions. Mechanical ventilation is one example. Mechanical ventilation (ventilators) are required for children with a variety of medical conditions, including severe neurological and respiratory conditions, and serious muscle weakness. Ventilators may be used to totally breathe for the child, or as a supplement for children who cannot breathe effectively.

Most ventilators work by providing air exchange through the use of pressure. Positive pressure ventilation machines are used to delivery air into the lungs, usually through the use of a tracheostomy tube. This is the most common and most portable method of artificial ventilation.

Negative pressure ventilation machines provide a vacuum around the child, and bring air into the lungs by pulling the chest wall outward (Haynie, et al., 1989). This type of ventilation does not require a tracheostomy (Haynie, et al., 1989).

Most state laws and nursing/medical practice standards require ventilator care to be provided only by a specially trained nurse or respiratory therapist. A comprehensive discussion of the care and management of children on ventilators is beyond the scope of this chapter. It is strongly recommended that assessment and care planning for a child with a ventilator be conducted individually, and implemented accordingly. Caution should be taken in caring for a ventilator-dependent child in a school setting. Properly trained personnel and appropriate equipment must be available at all times that the child is in school. Failure to provide such professional backup may have life-threatening consequences.

BIBLIOGRAPHY

Ahmann, E. (1986). *Home care for the high risk infant: A holistic guide to using technology.* Rockville, Aspen.

Andrews, M., & Nielson, D. (1988). Technology dependent children in the home. *Pediatric Nursing, 14*(2), 111-151.

Briggs, N. (1987). Selecting a pediatric home care program. *Pediatric Nursing, 13*(3), 191.

Caldwell, T., Todaro, A., Gates, A., & Pailet, J. (Eds.). (1989). *Community provider's guide: An information outline for working with children with special health needs.* New Orleans, LA: Children's Hospital.

Gadow, K. (1985). *Children on medication: A primer for school personnel.* Reston, VA: The Council for Exceptional Children.

Haddad, A. (1987). *High tech home care: A practical guide.* Rockville, MD: Aspen.

Hartsell, M., & Ward, J. (1985). Selecting equipment vendors for children on home care. *Maternal Child Nursing, 10*, 26-28.

Huddleston, K., & Palmer, K. (1990). A button for gastrostomy feedings. *Maternal and Child Nursing, 15*, 315-319.

Kaufman, J., & Hardy-Ribakow, D. (1987). Home care: A model of a comprehensive approach for technology assisted chronically ill children. *Journal of Pediatric Nursing, 2*(4), 244-249.

Nelson, C., & Hallgren, R. (1990). Gastrostomies: Indications, management and weaning. *Infants and Young Children, 2*(1), 66-74.

Reynolds, E., & Kirkland, S. (1989). Alternatives in gastrostomy management. *Journal of Enterostomal Therapy, 16*(3), 134-136.

Ritchie, P., & Greenburg, G. (1985). Guidelines for the administration of medication in day care centers. *Journal of Community Health Nursing, 2*(3), 145-149.

7

PROMOTING GOOD
HEALTH

Children with special health care needs spend an inordinate amount of time in doctor's offices and hospitals. This time is generally related to specific problems and treatments. However, basic health promotion needs common to all children frequently are not addressed.

Two factors contribute to this omission. First, many generalized pediatricians are not comfortable providing care to a child with special health care needs, preferring to refer these children to their more specialized colleagues. Secondly, many specialists who provide complex care to specific organ systems or for certain diseases do not deal with the overall needs of the child. Thus, the generic needs of the child are overlooked.

A similar pattern exists in the care provided by other disciplines. Traditional emphasis on problem identification and interventions directed toward problem resolution are not compatible with primary health care needs.

WHAT IS PRIMARY HEALTH CARE?

Primary health care encompasses routine health care (health histories, measurements, developmental and behavioral assessments, screening examinations, routine laboratory tests, and physical examinations), anticipatory guidance, and health education. The aim of primary care is to promote optimal health habits so disease does not occur, as well as to identify possible problems early.

ROUTINE HEALTH CARE

The American Academy of Pediatrics recommends preventive health care visits to a physician by 1 month of age and again at 2, 4, 6, 9, 12, 15, 18, and 24 months, with subsequent visits at 3 and 4 years (Blackman, 1990). During these visits, a health history is taken. This history provides valuable information regarding the child's general health and episodes of illness or accidents. Data such as height, weight, and head circumference serve as objective indicators of growth and often give the first warning of developmental delay.

Developmental assessments indicate progress toward developmental milestones. Behavioral assessments may clarify parental concerns, as well as serve as indicators of parent and child interactions. Combined information from these assessments provide information regarding the influence of a health problem on the child's general level of adaptive functioning. For example, Johnny has a cardiac condition. He shows irritability and fatigue after playing with his father before dinner. Johnny does not eat well at dinner and goes to sleep immediately afterward. Such behaviors may be caused by pre-dinner activities that are too strenuous for Johnny, given his tendency to tire easily. A change to more quiet play may lessen fatigue and improve eating behavior.

Screening examinations are done to identify problems early. Some examinations, such as those for vision and hearing, are routinely done on all children. Others, such as those for certain types of metabolic screening, are conducted if the child possesses specific risk factors.

Laboratory tests serve as an indicator of internal body functioning. Test results may indicate problems before they become noticeable. Common laboratory tests include hematocrit or hemoglobin and urinalysis.

Physical examinations are generally head to toe assessments of physical appearance. The techniques of observation, palpation, percussion, and auscultation are used to identify abnormal findings. Additional laboratory tests and procedures may be used for further evaluation.

The physical examination is an ideal time to inquire about parental concerns and questions. Many times, parents are concerned about observations or behaviors that are within normal limits. The care provider can use this opportunity to discuss the wide ranges of normal findings and prescribe medications or other interventions to resolve abnormal findings.

The physical examination also provides the opportunity to discuss normal sequences of growth and development. Many children with special health care needs show delays in some or all sectors of development. However, health care providers can alleviate much concern by pointing out the child's strengths, and progress toward the normal *sequence* of development.

This is also a good time to discuss future stages in growth and development and provide anticipatory guidance regarding the management of these stages. Many parents are unaware of normal growth and development trends. The situation becomes more complicated when a child has special health care needs that delay the sequence, for parents may attribute normal behaviors for a particular age to the underlying diagnosis rather than development. For example, a mother brought a child with a severe genetic problem into the office for an evaluation. The child was chronologically 4 years old, but was functioning at a 2-year-old level. The mother was very concerned with recent increases in her child's severe temper tantrums. She felt the behavior was a manifestation of the condition and feared that she would not be able to cope with such behaviors as the child became older. A subsequent comprehensive examination confirmed the care provider's initial impressions that the temper tantrum behavior had no cause other than that attributed to "the terrible twos." A lengthy discussion of growth and development sequences and measures to provide limits for behavior helped to resolve the parent's concern. Long-term followup confirmed that the temper tantrum behavior was short-lived.

When a family includes a child with special health care needs, anticipatory guidance should also include explorations of the family's concerns and perceptions about the child, care, social supports, and opportunities for respite. The health care provider can discuss the current status of the health problem and explain the effects the disease or disorder can have on current and subsequent growth and development. Early indicators of possible future problems can also be identified.

When a child has special health care needs, the constant responsibility for caregiving, especially if the therapeutic procedures are complex, is financially and personally draining. Health care providers must acknowledge these stressors and assist the family in coping with them, to the degree the family desires. Finally, anticipatory guidance provides the basis for subsequent health education. Educational topics relate to primary preventive measures and strategies for health promotion. They center around immunizations; safety; rest and sleep; exercise; dental health; feeding, fluid, and elimination; parent and child interactions, and optimal growth and development.

IMMUNIZATIONS

Routine immunizations provide acquired immunity against many formerly devastating childhood diseases and are a part of primary health care. Some parents, however, must be educated that medical care is not just for illness, and that children should receive preventive care to promote wellness.

The American Academy of Pediatrics has recently updated its recommended schedule for immunizations of healthy infants and children (American Academy of Pediatrics, 1991). (See Table 7-1.) While these recommendations are for well children, they are also generally applicable for children with special health needs (American Academy of Pediatrics, 1991). Sometimes, immunization schedules may be altered due to frequent illnesses. The child's individual physician will make the final determinations, but will generally weigh the potential risk from the immunizations against the potential effect of the illness.

Immunodeficient and immunosuppressed children also need immunizations, but may need some modifications in schedule. Children with congenital disorders of immune function should not receive live bacterial and viral vaccines, but may receive inactive vaccine and immune globulins instead (American Academy of Pediatrics, 1991).

Children with HIV infections and AIDS should receive the measles, mumps, and rubella vaccination (MMR), the diptheria, tetanus and pertussis vaccine (DTP), the Haemophilus B influenza immunization, and the pneumococcal vaccine. Inactivated polio vaccine should be given instead of oral polio vaccine (American Academy of Pediatrics, 1991). (See Table 7-2.)

SAFETY

Accidents are one of the leading causes of death in children in the United States. Children with special health care needs, especially if they suffer from reduced coordination, strength or endurance, are at even greater risk.

TABLE 7-1. Recommended Schedule For Immunization Of Healthy Infants And Children.

RECOMMENDED AGE	IMMUNIZATION	COMMENTS
2 months	DTP, HbCV, and OPV	DTP protects against diphtheria, tetanus, and pertussis (whooping cough); OPV stands for oral polio vaccine; HbCV is a new immunization which protects against hemophilus influenza (H-flu)
4 months	DTP, HbCV, and OPV	
6 months	DTP, HbCV	
15 months	MMR, HbCV	MMR is a combination vaccine which protects against measles, mumps, and rubella; tuberculin testing may also be done at this visit; if a child has allergies to eggs, special desensitization precautions are indicated in the administration of MMR (Levine & Lavi, 1991).
15-18 months	DTP, OPV	
4-6 years	DTP and OPV	At or before school entry.
11-12 years	MMR	Required at entry to middle school or junior high school, unless the child has already had a second dose.
14-16 years	Td	For tetanus and diphtheria; repeat every 10 years throughout life.

Adapted from: American Academy of Pediatrics, (1991). *Report of the committee on infectious diseases.* American Academy of Pediatrics, p. 17.

All professionals should share the responsibility to provide safe environments for children, as well as to teach parents and others about safety measures. Special areas of concern include child safety restraints in cars; smoke detectors (especially when specialized electrical equipment or oxygen is in use); prevention of burns (especially with hot water); prevention of falls; prevention of aspiration from ingestion of small toys or food (especially in a child with oral motor problems); prevention of poisoning (especially from plants in the environment); and first aid for injuries.

Professionals in mainstreaming situations must also realize that situations that would be safe for many children may be dangerous to a child with special health care needs. For example, if a child had limitations in balance due to musculo-skeletal problems, the child may not be able to safely use all playground equipment without assistance.

TABLE 7-2. Recommendations For Routine Immunization Of HIV-Infected Children In The United States.

VACCINE	KNOWN ASYMPTOMATIC HIV INFECTION	SYMPTOMATIC HIV INFECTION
DTP	Yes	Yes
OPV	No	No
IPV	Yes	Yes
MMR	Yes	Yes
Hemophilus B	Yes	Yes
Pneumococcal	Yes	Yes
Influenza	Should be considered	Yes

DTP = Diphtheria and tetanus toxoids and pertussis vaccine
OPV = Oral poliovirus vaccine
IPV = Inactivated poliovirus vaccine
MMR = Live virus measles, mumps, and rubella

Reprinted with permission from *Report of the committee on infectious diseases.* Copyright ® 1991. American Academy of Pediatrics.

REST AND SLEEP

All children need adequate rest and sleep to replenish and rebuild their bodies after play. Many children with special health care needs require more frequent rest periods or additional sleep.

An assessment of sleep/awake patterns is a helpful tool in evaluating the adequacy of rest and sleep. Not only does objective documentation of behavior provide parents with helpful insight, but a weekly activity log can also provide clues to behavioral interventions. Techniques such as a soothing bath or a quiet reading time before bed may assist a child in quieting behavior to prepare for sleep. Caregiving procedures and medication administration can often be scheduled around rest periods.

EXERCISE

Just as rest and sleep are important, so is activity. Large and small muscle use is important for optimal growth and development.

Children with special health care needs may require modifications in life-style to facilitate adequate exercise. For example, adaptive equipment can enhance mobility and endurance. Developmental stimulation or therapy can be integrated into play activity to simultaneously accomplish goals of therapy, exercise, and fun.

Be sure to include the child's physician in planning for a child's exercise regimen. Some diagnoses adversely affect the child's exercise tolerance or types of activities that may be pursued safely. Frequent periods of inactivity due to illness or hospitalizations must be considered in overall exercise plans.

DENTAL HEALTH

Dental disease can be related to poor care, trauma, or a variety of congenital or acquired diseases. Dental caries can result from poor diet or improper dental care. Many children with developmental disabilities also have gum problems, often attributed to poor oral hygiene. Some medications such as Dilantin can result in overgrowth of the gum. Neuromuscular problems of the head and neck can contribute to abnormal posturing responses, oral defensiveness, difficulty swallowing, tongue thrusting, and prolonged gag and bite reflexes. (Zelle & Coyner, 1983). These factors can affect feeding and dental hygiene.

To promote dental health, parents should be instructed in appropriate oral hygiene for their infant. A visit to the dentist should be made while the child is still very young. Because many children with special health care needs provide special challenges for dental care, it is helpful to identify a dentist who is interested in providing the care. Preventive care can do much to avoid later problems.

FEEDING, FLUID, AND ELIMINATION

Many children with special health care needs have special requirements related to feeding, fluid and elimination. Some children have special dietary requirements to compensate for disease or disability. These requirements may relate to dietary restrictions, supplements, or external methods of administration (e.g., gastrostomy tubes). For example, children with spasticity or hypertonicity require additional calories for growth. Children with Down syndrome, hydrocephalus, or spina bifida may have a tendency toward excessive weight gain and may require fewer calories for growth. Children with a tendency toward constipation may need increased bulk and fluids. Children with urinary tract diseases or disorders may need additional fluids. Children with severe cardiac conditions or gastrointestinal problems may need special formulas. Children with poor sucking abilities, aggravated gag reflexes or gastrointestinal reflux may need additional interdisciplinary interventions in addition to dietary modifications.

Because children with special health care needs often need modifications in feeding, fluid, and elimination practices, an interdisciplinary assessment is recommended. The group, in concert with the family and the child's physician, can then develop an individualized plan of care designed to meet current needs and avoid future problems.

PARENT-CHILD INTERACTIONS

A child's illness or disability can adversely affect the development of optimal parent-child interactions. The phenomenon is complex and encompasses the family's expectations, responses to illness, cultural values and beliefs, and coping strategies.

When a child's illness involves complex and time-consuming treatment protocols, stress becomes a factor in the relationship between the parent and the child. Eye-to-eye contact, verbal and nonverbal responses of both the parent and child, and varying perceptions of family members should be evaluated (Steele, 1988).

OPTIMAL GROWTH AND DEVELOPMENT

Many children with health problems suffer from subsequent developmental delay or disability. To avoid such delays as much as possible, the interdisciplinary team should promote growth and development, attempt to identify early signs of delay, and plan early intervention strategies designed to minimize the adverse effects of the disease or condition.

Developmental screening tests should be an integral part of primary health care. Since one-time results can be misleading, longitudinal screening is preferred (Steele, 1988). Based on the results of these screening tests, intervention strategies and stimulation activities can be developed.

It is important to remember that a child's self concept is very tightly interwoven with physical and mental abilities and independence. Normalization of growth and development experiences, to the degree possible, facilitates optimal psychosocial development.

Increasing awareness of health promotion and primary prevention will also promote optimal growth and development. As professionals become more accustomed to addressing family and child strengths, a more holistic approach to care will evolve.

BIBLIOGRAPHY

Gunnip, A., Roberson, C., Meredith, J., Bull, M., Stroup, K., & Branson, M. (1987). Car seats: Helping parents do it right. *Journal of Pediatric Health Care, 1*(4), 190-195.

Richardson, S. (1988). Child health promotion practices. *Journal of Pediatric Health Care, 2*(2), 73-78.

Sharts-Engel, N. (1990). Pertussis vaccine: Safety update. *Maternal Child Nursing, 15*(5), 293.

U.S. Department of Health and Human Resources. (1990). *Healthy people: National health promotion and disease prevention objectives* (DHHS Publication No. PHS 91-50212). Washington, DC: Author.

8

WHEN A CHILD IS SICK

Communicable diseases are one of the leading causes of illness in children. This is true even if the child's primary diagnosis is a chronic or a medically complex disorder.

This chapter will contain a description of some basic concepts of communicable disease control and natural history of disease; the professional's role in disease prevention, including universal precautions; recognition of symptoms of communicable disease; recommended exclusion and readmission guidelines; and a brief summary of specific conditions that may be seen in preschool children.

BASIC CONCEPTS OF INFECTION CONTROL

To control communicable disease, one must first understand how it occurs. The development of a communicable disease requires the presence of three factors: an agent, a host, and a supportive environment.

Agent

The agent is an infectious organism capable of causing a disease. The organism can normally be found in a person or in the environment. Agents vary greatly in their strength, mode of transmission, point of entry and exit from the host, and harmful effects. Specific organisms cause specific diseases. For example, chickenpox is always caused by the varicella-zoster virus.

Host

The host is the susceptible person who provides the suitable living conditions for the agent, thereby promoting the development of disease. Host characteristics such as age, general health status, fatigue, physiological characteristics, and immunity influence the degree to which the host can resist the agent.

Environment

External environments can also influence the development of disease. Physical characteristics, such as the climate and places of school and play, influence the types of organisms to which a person may become exposed. Socioeconomic factors such as housing and family financial status are statistically related to exposure to harmful agents. Practices of hygiene, diet, exercise, behavior, preventive health care, and social interactions are key factors in disease prevention and early detection.

Interaction of Agent, Host, and Environment

The interaction of agent, host, and environment determines communicable disease spread. Infection control requires identification of factors promoting the spread of specific organisms and interruption of key factors in the interaction of this triad.

NATURAL HISTORY OF DISEASE

Each communicable disease goes through an individualized sequence known as the natural history of the disease. Although the natural history varies from one disease to another, it is always consistent for a specific disease. This uniformity facilitates diagnosis and treatment.

In most communicable diseases, the agent (organism) is spread from an infected person to a potential host by a method of transmission specific to that organism. Most commonly, communicable diseases are transmitted through droplets of water that are spread during speech, or from direct or indirect exposure to body fluids such as nasal discharge, saliva, feces, and urine.

At first, the new host may not feel ill, but the pathogenic organisms are growing in the body. This period between initial exposure and the appearance of the first symptoms is the incubation period.

During the next stage, the prodromal period, subtle symptoms may be noted. This is the time when one may say, "I feel like I am coming down with something." Toward the end of this period, fever, rash, or other symptoms may occur.

The next stage is characterized by objective clinical signs and subjective symptoms. Signs and symptoms generally worsen for a few days to a few weeks, peak, and then disappear.

The final stage is convalescence. During this period, the affected individual gradually regains previous health and energy.

PROFESSIONAL'S ROLE IN DISEASE PREVENTION

The professional's responsibilities in disease prevention are two-fold: primary prevention and early identification.

Primary Prevention

Primary prevention includes actions that keep a disease from occurring in the first place. Several effective preventative strategies have been found.

Health Education

Teaching about good health practices can increase the incidence of these positive behaviors.

Immunizations

The professional has a critical role in helping to assure that a child receives appropriate immunizations. This is usually accomplished through tracking of immunization records. Immunizations help the body to develop antibodies which protect against certain childhood diseases.

Handwashing

Proper handwashing is one of the most effective methods of primary prevention. Its importance cannot be overemphasized (Anderson, 1988). Proper technique includes consistent and thorough washing before and after each contact with a child, use of the bathroom, or contact with food and equipment, even if gloves were worn.

When handwashing, use soap and running water. Vigorously rub your hands to provide additional friction for germ and dirt removal. Be sure to include under the fingernails, between the fingers, the back of the hands, and around the wrists. Remove jewelry so underlying skin surfaces can be cleansed. Rinse well and dry hands with a paper towel (Centers for Disease Control, 1985).

Universal Precautions

In response to increased rates of hepatitis and human immunodeficiency virus (HIV) infections, the Centers for Disease Control recommended that special precautions be used for all blood and body fluids. The underlying rationale of universal precautions is that all persons should be treated as potentially communicable, and appropriate precautions should be taken.

Practically, this means that gloves should be worn whenever contact with blood or blood-contaminated fluids is possible (Centers for Disease Control, 1987). These guidelines refer to blood, semen, and cerebrospinal, synovial, vaginal, and pericardial fluids. Gloves should also be worn when performing procedures such as finger and heel sticks, tracheostomy suctioning, and rinsing of used instruments (American Academy of Pediatrics, 1988). A common error made by staff is not changing gloves before handling another child. This practice may protect the caregiver, but it does not prevent infection spread from one child to another.

Gloves usage also pertains to cleaning up an area that may have been in contact with blood or blood contaminated fluids. Blot the spill with disposable towels to reduce the amount. Throw away all contaminated materials, including gloves, in a doubled plastic bag labeled "Caution: contaminated materials." (Check with your local health department for other disposal regulations.) Remove gloves, avoiding contact with the contaminated outside part of the gloves. Dispose of the gloves in the plastic bag.

Next, apply new gloves. Clean the spill area with a 1:10 household bleach solution (1 part household bleach mixed with 10 parts of water), made fresh daily. Carefully remove the gloves and dispose in the plastic bag. Wash your hands.

Although the AIDS virus has been found in other body fluids, contact with these fluids is not considered to be high risk. Thus, handwashing only is recommended for contact with urine, stool, vomitus, tears, nasal secretions, oral secretions, and diaper changing (American Academy of Pediatrics, 1988).

Universal precautions should be practiced in all high risk areas, or when the possibility of infection spread through direct contact or care is high. Communities with lower disease rates may temper the guidelines (American Academy of Pediatrics, 1991).

General Environmental Infection Control Precautions

Infection control on a routine as well as emergency basis is critical to prevent disease transmission. Each school should practice infection control precautions in personal hygiene, food preparation, handling and storage, diapering and toileting, insect control, cleaning and disinfecting, and environmental safety and sanitation monitoring. Guidelines are available through local health departments. The American Academy of Pediatrics also provides recommendations for care of children in day care, including those with special health care needs (American Academy of Pediatrics, 1991).

Early Identification

Secondary prevention refers to early identification of signs and symptoms. Early identification is important so an individual can receive proper care and complications can be avoided.

Initial Symptoms

Early symptoms of infection occur several days before the child becomes noticeably ill. These symptoms may include malaise, listlessness, headache, loss of appetite, and lightheadedness. Obviously, a child who is very young or developmentally delayed may not be able to describe these subtle symptoms. Most often, they are manifested to the caregiver by a change in the usual behavior of the child.

Suspicious Symptoms

Symptoms warranting further action include unexpected rise in body temperature; yellow or greenish discharge; a productive cough; skin lesions (sores) or tenderness.

When suspicious symptoms are noted, additional investigation is indicated. Note and document signs and symptoms in writing. For example, if the child has a rash, describe the size, shape, distribution, and severity. Note how long the child has experienced the symptoms and if they are local or generalized throughout the entire body. Investigate whether the child has recently (within the last month) been in contact with another person with similar symptoms. Conversations with other professionals and with the family may contribute valuable information. Remember, the professional's job is to attempt to determine whether a communicable condition exists. It is the physician's role to make the diagnosis.

Interventions

Initial interventions relate to the safety and comfort of the affected child. If ill, the child is probably not interested in regular classroom activity. For the sake of the child, the teacher responsible for classroom management, and the health of others, the child should be moved to a quiet location. Assure ongoing adult supervision.

Assure that the Child is not in Immediate Danger

Be sure that the child is having no difficulty with basic body functions such as breathing. These problems are highly unlikely, but if present they require emergency action.

Contact the Parent

The parent should be notified of any illness in the child and included in any action plans. The parent is also an excellent source of additional information regarding exposure or health habits that may assist the physician in diagnosis. If the parent cannot be contacted, school personnel must assume responsibility for providing additional care for the child until contact is made.

Determine if the Child has an Elevated Temperature

Most preschools restrict temperature-taking to the axillary route. A child is considered to have a fever if the axillary temperature is above 100 degrees Fahrenheit (Wong & Whaley, 1990). (See Table 8-1 for a description of the method of axillary temperature.)

TABLE 8-1. Measurement Of An Axillary Temperature.

This procedure can be used safely to measure temperature in preschool and school-age children. Take an axillary temperature if the child feels warm to the touch or if the child's behavior is unusual for that child.

1. Explain the procedure to the child;
2. Grasp the thermometer at the end opposite the bulb. Quickly shake the thermometer to bring the mercury level to below 96 degrees Fahrenheit;
3. Position the thermometer under the axilla; the silver end of the thermometer should rest in the middle of the child's armpit for the most accurate measurement;
4. Hold the child's arm firmly next to the body; leave the thermometer in place for 5-10 minutes;
5. Remove the thermometer and praise the child for cooperating;
6. Read and record the time and temperature readings.

Schools' guidelines for managing temperature elevations also vary. While many schools have written guidelines regarding doses of Acetaminophen for children of varying weights and ages, others feel elevated temperatures are the body's way of fighting infection. Be sure to determine organizational policy in advance of need.

If medications are given, follow the guidelines for medication administration discussed in Chapter 6. Be cautioned that aspirin and aspirin products should never be given to children without the doctor's instructions, especially if the child is suffering from a viral illness.

A sponge bath is often used to gradually lower an elevated temperature. It is critical that the child's temperature is not lowered too abruptly or serious consequences could result. Use lukewarm water rather than cold water. Never use ice water or alcohol.

Exclusion Guidelines

School personnel must be concerned with the overall health of children in their care, as well as the health of the individual. Thus, for the potential good of all, there are times when an ill child must be removed from the classroom setting. Although these guidelines do not apply to children with minor illnesses, the American Academy of Pediatrics (1991) does recommend temporary exclusion for the following conditions:

- The illness prevents the child from participating comfortably in program activities.
- The illness results in a greater care need than the child care staff can provide without compromising the health and safety of the other children.
- The child has any of the following conditions: fever, unusual lethargy, irritability, persistent crying, difficult breathing, or other signs of possible severe illness.
- Diarrhea (defined as an increased number of stools compared with the child's normal pattern, with increased stool water and/or decreased form) that is not contained by diapers or toilet use.
- Vomiting two or more times in the previous 24 hours unless the vomiting is determined to be due to a noncommunicable condition and the child is not in danger of dehydration.
- Mouth sores associated with an inability of the child to control his/her saliva, unless the child's physician or local health department authority states that the child is noninfectious.

- Rash with fever or behavior change until a physician has determined the illness not to be a communicable disease.

- Purulent conjunctivitis (defined as pink or red conjunctiva with white or yellow eye discharge, often with matted eyelids after sleep and eye pain or redness of the eyelids or skin surrounding the eye), until examined by a physician and approved for readmission, with or without treatment.

- Tuberculosis, until the child's physician or local health department authority states the child is noninfectious.

- Impetigo, until 24 hours after treatment has been initiated.

- Streptococcal pharyngitis, until 24 hours after treatment has been initiated, and until the child has been afebrile for 24 hours.

- Head lice (pediculosis) until the morning after the first treatment.

- Scabies, until after treatment has been completed.

- Varicella, until the sixth day after onset of rash or sooner if all lesions have dried and crusted.

- Pertussis (which is confirmed by laboratory or suspected based on symptoms of the illness or because of cough onset within 14 days of having face-to-face contact with a person in a household or classroom who has a laboratory-confirmed case of pertussis), until 5 days of appropriate antibiotic therapy (currently erythromycin) has been completed (total course of treatment is 14 days).

- Mumps, until 9 days after onset of parotid gland swelling.

- Hepatitis A virus infection until one week after onset of illness and jaundice, if present, has disappeared or until passive immunoprophylaxis (immune serumglobulin) has been administered to appropriate children and staff in the program, as directed by the responsible health department. (pp. 70-71).

Unless one of the conditions just discussed exists, the American Academy of Pediatrics (1991) says a child should not automatically be excluded from school for:

asymptomatic secretion of an enteropathogen; nonpurulent conjunctivitis (defined as pink conjunctiva with a clear, watery eye discharge and without fever, eye pain or eyelid redness); rash without fever and without behavior change; cytomegalovirus infection; hepatitis B virus carrier state; and HIV infection. (p. 71)

Likewise, children with mild or moderately severe colds, croup, bronchitis, pneumonia, and ear infections do not need to be excluded from child care (American Academy of Pediatrics, 1991).

Readmission Guidelines

The following are recommendations for re-entry into school following an illness.

1. Significant improvement in overall health status has been made, as agreed by both parents and school personnel.
2. The child's physician determines re-entry is safe for the child and classmates.
3. If the illness is part of an epidemic, state and local guidelines regarding testing and treatment must be followed.

Report to the Health Department

State laws often require schools to report certain diseases to the local health department. This action facilitates disease follow-up and national reporting. Check with the local health department for specific guidelines.

Report to the Parents

Parents should be encouraged to report to the school when a child is kept from school because of a contagious disease. Whether a disease is reported by a parent or noted by staff, all parents should then be notified of the presence of a communicable disease in the school. Written notification should include the name of the disease, prevention, incubation period, period of greatest communicability, methods of spread, early signs and symptoms, possible consequences, and recommended courses of action (American Academy of Pediatrics, 1987). Since parents are alerted to early indications of disease, they can detect future illness early. Keeping children home during the prodromal period (which is often the most contagious period) contributes to overall communicable disease control.

Parental notification also provides essential information in case the child with special health care needs is particularly at risk. For example, a child with an altered immune system due to illness or certain medications may find a case of chickenpox to be potentially life-threatening. Exposure warrants early medical intervention.

EMPLOYEE HEALTH

To minimize the spread of infection from employees to children in their care, staff should be expected to conform to similar guidelines. Physical examinations, screening tests, and staff exclusion/readmission policies should be made a part of all orientation programs as well as ongoing personnel policies.

SPECIFIC CONDITIONS

It should be emphasized that diagnosis of a condition is within the responsibility of the child's physician. However, school personnel frequently desire a reference to obtain additional information regarding specific conditions. The American Academy of Pediatrics, the American Public Health Association and the Centers for Disease Control are excellent sources of reference materials. (See the Appendix for addresses of these organizations.)

Although there are numerous communicable diseases, some are more prevalent in the preschool years than others. Table 8-2 provides a summary of communicable diseases that are most commonly found in preschool group setting.

These summaries provide an overview of the agent, incubation time, communicable period, transmission, and symptoms of some of the most common communicable diseases noted in preschoolers. It should be emphasized, however, that the use of the general infection precautions discussed earlier in this chapter will do much to decrease the incidence of all of these diseases. It is much easier to prevent infection than provide care for the child who is sick.

BIBLIOGRAPHY

Andersen, R., Bale, J., Blackman, J., & Murph, J. (1986). *Infections in children: A sourcebook for educators and child care providers*. Rockville, MD: Aspen.

Benenson, A. (1990). *Control of communicable diseases in man* (15th ed.). Washington, DC: American Public Health Association.

Taylor, J., & Taylor, W. (1989). *Communicable disease and young children in group settings*. Boston: College-Hill Press.

TABLE 8-2. Summary Of Communicable Diseases.

DISEASE	AGENT	INCUBATION	COMMUNICABLE PERIOD	TRANSMISSION	SYMPTOMS	REMARKS
Chickenpox (Herpes Zoster; Varicella; Shingles)	Virus	2-3 weeks	1-5 days before rash; no more than 6 days after first vesicles	Direct contact with vesicle fluid, soiled articles, or droplets from respiratory tract	Sudden onset; slight fever; malaise; mild constitutional symptoms, followed by eruption of lesions; followed by fluid filled blisters for 3-4 days; ending with scab	Very communicable; lesions, blisters and scabbed sores can exist at the same time; lesions are most common on covered parts of the body
Conjunctivitis (Pink Eye)	Bacteria	24-72 hours	Throughout course of infection	Contact with discharge from conjunctiva or upper respiratory tract, or objects contaminated by those discharges	Tearing and irritation of conjunctiva; lid swelling, discharge; sensitivity to light	Most common in preschoolers
Cytomegalovirus (CMV)	Virus	May be acquired during birth, but show no symptoms for up to 3 months after delivery	Virus may be excreted for 5-6 years	Direct/indirect contact with membranes or secretions; blood; urine	Usually no symptoms; may show signs of severe infection of central nervous system or liver	Most serious in early infancy; many apparently healthy children in day care have CMV in urine or saliva
Giardiasis	Protozoa (a cyst in the inactive form)	5-25 days	Entire period of infection	Hand to mouth transfer of cysts from stools of infected person	Chronic pale, greasy diarrhea; abdominal cramping; fatigue; weight loss	Frequently found in day care centers; carriers may be asymptomatic
Hepatitis	Several viruses	Hepatitis A: 15-50 days;	Hepatitis A: A week before infection to one week after appearance of jaundice	Hepatitis A: Fecal/oral route; direct contact	Hepatitis A: sudden onset with fever, lack of appetite, nausea, abdominal pain; jaundice follows in a few days	Hepatitis A: Common in day care; severity increases with age; infections in infants may be asymptomatic

(continued)

179

TABLE 8-2. *(continued)*

DISEASE	AGENT	INCUBATION	COMMUNICABLE PERIOD	TRANSMISSION	SYMPTOMS	REMARKS
		Hepatitis B: 45-180 days	Hepatitis B: From several weeks before symptoms until weeks after symptoms; may be a carrier for years	Hepatitis B: Contact with infected blood; saliva, and vaginal fluids; semen	Hepatitis B: Lack of appetite; nausea, vomiting and later jaundice	Hepatitis B: May be present but asymptomatic in young children; HB vaccine available to prevent this type of hepatitis
Measles (Rubeola, hard measles; red measles)	Virus	1-2 weeks before rash to 4 days after the rash appears	Communicable from before fever to 4 days after rash	Direct contact with nasal or throat secretions or freshly contaminated objects	Fever, conjunctivitis, cough, Koplik spots; rash appears on 3rd day—usually starting on face	Easily spread; very common in pre-school populations; immunization available; potentially serious for ill or young children
Meningitis (Viral)	Several viruses	Incubation varies by specific virus	Communicability varies with specific virus	Direct contact with respiratory droplets or excretions of infected person, or objects contaminated by these secretions	Symptoms vary by specific type of virus; usually sudden fever and central nervous system symptoms; may have rash	Symptoms last 10 days with residual symptoms for a year or more
Meningitis (Bacterial)	Various bacteria	2-10 days	Until organisms are not found in discharge	Direct contact with respiratory droplets or excretions of an infected person or objects contaminated by these secretions	Sudden onset of fever; severe headache; stiff neck; rash	Early detection and treatment necessary to prevent death
Mumps	Virus	2-3 weeks	6 days before until 9 days after onset of illness	Direct contact with respiratory droplets or saliva of infected person	Fever, swelling and tenderness of one or more salivary glands	Meningitis occurs frequently; Vaccine available

Disease	Causative Agent	Incubation Period	Period of Communicability	Mode of Transmission	Symptoms	Comments
Pediatric AIDS	Virus	Unknown	Unknown	Contact with blood and blood contaminated fluids and objects; sexual contact with semen and vaginal fluids	Early symptoms are nonspecific: loss of appetite; chronic diarrhea; fatigue; symptoms progress to opportunistic infections and central nervous system symptoms	Use universal precautions
Pediculosis (Lice)	Lice Adult, (larvae or nits)	Eggs hatch in a week; sexual maturity is reached 8–10 days after hatching	Communicable as long as eggs and lice are alive on person or clothing	Direct contact with infected person or indirect contact with contaminated objects	Itching and excoriation of infected head and body parts	Common in school children; Check with physician regarding use of over-the-counter products; some are not recommended for infants and young children
Ringworm	Fungus	4–10 days	Until lesions are gone and fungus is no longer on contaminated objects	Direct or indirect contact with infected persons or contaminated objects	Lesions appear flat, spreading, and ring shaped; outer ring may be filled with pus or fluid; inside may be dry and scaly or moist and crusty	Infected children should be excluded from common swimming pools
Rubella	Virus	2–3 weeks	From one week before to one week after onset of rash	Droplet spread or direct/indirect contact with objects soiled with nasal secretions, blood, urine or feces	Symptoms may range from no symptoms to cold-like symptoms such as low grade fever, malaise, and runny nose; not all infections have a rash; if it does exist, it usually starts on the face, and spreads to trunk and extremities	Easily spread; high incidence in pre-school populations; immunization available; resembles measles

(continued)

TABLE 8-2. (continued)

DISEASE	AGENT	INCUBATION	COMMUNICABLE PERIOD	TRANSMISSION	SYMPTOMS	REMARKS
Scabies	Mite	2-6 weeks in person with no exposure; 1-4 days after re-exposure	Until mites and eggs are killed; usually 1-2 courses of treatment, one week apart	Skin to skin contact, or contact with recently infected undergarments or bed clothes	Intense itching of head, neck, palms, soles in infants; may also involve other body creases	In persons with reduced resistance, infection will be generalized; check with physician prior to use of over-the-counter medications, because some are not recommended for infants and young children

9

EMERGENCIES

No one likes to think that an emergency will happen. Especially when the emergency involves illness or injury of a young child. Unfortunately, such events do occur. These situations may involve life-threatening emergencies, or non-life threatening situations requiring medical attention.

It must be an unwritten rule that "emergencies happen at inopportune times." Any preschool teacher will confirm that emergencies occur late in the day (when some of the staff have already left) or at the most hectic time of the school day. A corollary is "when emergencies occur, it is usually difficult to contact the parents." Often, the parents are not home to answer the phone. Sometimes, the phone number has been recently disconnected or changed.

Preparation includes a school-wide plan for preventing, recognizing, and dealing with emergencies. It also includes training to prepare child care workers to recognize and manage emergency situations quickly and appropriately. Each center should have written policies and procedures regarding handling emergencies. Individualized standing orders, developed in conjunction with the child's physician and the family, may be indicated.

This chapter includes general emergency planning for children with special health care needs, recognizing and responding to major emergencies and general managing non-life-threatening emergencies. Due to the necessity of modifying care to meet the special health care needs of each child, these recommendations do not indicate an exclusive course of action. Variations, depending on individual situations, may be appropriate.

EMERGENCY PLANNING

All preschools must be equipped to handle emergencies related to fire, naturally occurring events, and routine accidents. While all preschool programs must do some planning for emergencies, there are several special considerations when the program cares for young children with special health care needs.

Fire

Potential or actual fires are the most common reasons for emergency evacuation of a center. When children with special health care needs are in the school, evacuation plans must include methods of removing large numbers of children who will need assistance in moving quickly to a place of safety. Several children can be transported in a rolling crib or in a wagon. These devices should be designed to provide back supports and security straps for older children and fit easily through doors. The use of such cribs or wagons provide a fast, efficient method of evacuation.

Special precautions against fire must be taken if oxygen is being administered within the school facility. Signs should be posted to warn of the presence of oxygen in the area. Cigarette smoking, candles, and other sources of fire should be prohibited in the area. Similar precautions should be taken on the school bus if oxygen is being transported.

Falls

Children with neurological or musculo-skeletal problems are at even greater risk for falls than children without these health problems. Limited mobility and poor balance can contribute directly to falls or limit the child's ability to move quickly to avoid an accident. School personnel should take these factors into consideration when selecting playground equipment and designing the physical environment of the school building and grounds.

Bleeding

An increasing number of children have conditions such as HIV infection and hepatitis that may be transmitted by contact with affected blood or objects that have come in contact with affected blood. For that reason, all schools should have nonsterile gloves readily available in emergency carts, classrooms, lunchrooms, and playground areas. In fact, many child care workers keep an extra set of gloves in a coat pocket at all times. Gloves should be used in all cases in which contact with blood or blood-contaminated objects may occur. Following use, these gloves should be discarded in accordance with universal infection control procedures. (Refer to Chapter 8 for further information about infection control measures.)

Bus Safety

If your school provides bus transportation for preschoolers with special health care needs, both the bus driver and an adult rider should be certified in first aid and pediatric cardiopulmonary resuscitation. If the children require tracheostomies or ventilators, the bus driver and adult rider should receive special training in related emergency procedures.

All buses should use approved infant and child safety car seats. Additionally, it is strongly recommended that each bus be equipped with a cellular telephone or citizen-band radio to assure access to the emergency medical services system in the event of accident or emergency.

ESTABLISHING EMERGENCY RESPONSE NETWORKS

When your program cares for children with special health needs, the network of community agencies involved in their care must be expanded. Community fire, ambulance, and police units should be notified in writing that the facility cares for young children. Provide the agency with the exact address and location of the center. Also notify them of the children's hours of attendance, special needs, and anticipated types of emergency assistance that may be needed. Frequently, emergency medical services units will recommend that a decal indicating the presence of an individual in need of special assistance be placed on the window.

When children are dependent on electrical equipment (such as that used for tracheostomy suctioning), the emergency medical services system should be notified in writing that a cessation of electricity to the area may create a medical emergency. The electrical utilities company should also be notified of the need to maintain electricity to the center. Personnel at the electrical company should be requested to notify the center of voluntary electrical shutdown. They should also be requested to restore electricity as soon as possible in the event of an unexpected outage. Each school should also purchase portable electrical generators and power cords to supply all emergency requirements on the school grounds and in the school buses.

Similarly, the telephone company should be notified of the presence of children with special health care needs, especially those with high technology equipment. Request that your center receive a priority rating for re-establishment of service so that emergency assistance can be readily requested when needed. Some centers prefer to have a cellular phone as an emergency backup.

Providing Emergency Directions

Too often, delay in reaching a child due to inadequate directions has resulted in death or avoidable, permanent disability. Thus, a critical part of establishing an emergency response network is providing comprehensive and accurate directions for emergency medical services system teams to use when locating the school.

The directions to the school must include not only the school's address, but directions from a nearby landmark or major intersection. Be sure your school has adequate outside signs so that the location can be easily identified from the street. Notify the emergency medical services (911 in most areas) of the exact location of the classrooms or programs housing children with special health care needs as well as the most direct method of access.

As a precaution, emergency response information should be posted next to all telephones throughout the center. It is amazingly difficult for a person making an emergency telephone call to remember this type of information. Post emergency telephone numbers for 911 or equivalent emergency medical services system teams, fire, police, and poison control centers. In addition, list the principal's number and that of the school nurse, if one is available.

EMERGENCY CONTACT CARDS

It is important for schools to gather comprehensive intake information regarding the child's medical problems, possible complications related to the diagnosis, and appropriate responses. (Figure 9-1 shows a sample emergency card.) Information should be shared with center staff and included in emergency planning. Anticipatory training should also be completed to enhance emergency responses.

Figure 9-1. Emergency contact card.

Child's Name: _____ Date of Birth _____
Address: _____ Sex: _____
Phone _____
Religion _____ Ethnic Origin _____
Mother's Name _____ Father's Name _____
Mother's Address _____ Father's Address _____
Home Telephone _____ Home Telephone _____
Work Address: _____ Work Address: _____
Work Telephone _____ Work Telephone _____
Work Hours _____ Work Hours: _____
Primary Language _____ Primary Language _____

Child's Diagnosis:
Special Concerns/Needs (Including allergies)
Current Medications: (List each medication and dose)
EMERGENCY CONTACT PERSON:
ADDRESS: TELEPHONE:
PHYSICIAN/CLINIC/HOSPITAL: TELEPHONE:
ADDRESS:

EMERGENCY EQUIPMENT VENDOR (IF INDICATED):
May the Center call another physician if unable to contact the above:
No _____ Yes _____
If so, do you have a preference?

_____
      (Doctor)   (Phone)
Persons Permitted to Remove the Child From the Program
(Names and phone numbers)

_____
_____

Other Emergency Contacts:

_____
(Name)   (Address)   (Phone)   (Relationship)
I hereby certify the above persons may remove the child from the school
in case of accident or illness.

_____
              (Signature and Date)

_____
              (Witness and Date)

I hereby certify the school principal or designee can authorize emergency
medical/nursing evaluation and treatment of my child

_____
              (Signature and Date)

_____
              (Witness and Date)

Dates of Update: (Updates At Least Every 6 Months)

To facilitate planning, an emergency contact card should be completed for each child. The card should be printed on heavy paper so it can withstand repeated handling. It should be placed in an easily accessible location in the classroom and taken with the teacher when the child goes out of the school on a field trip or other excursion. A duplicate up-to-date contact card should also be kept in the school van, if the child is transported to and from school each day. Parents should be told to report changes in telephone numbers and emergency contacts. Cards should be updated quarterly and emergency home contact numbers should be tested periodically to determine if they are still accurate.

EMERGENCY CARTS

Each school classroom should have a small first aid kit (easily available at local drugstores) to handle routine first aid needs such as cuts and bruises. However, each school that houses children with special health care needs should also have one or more larger emergency carts. These carts will contain emergency materials necessary in providing basic first aid and breathing support until an emergency medical services team can arrive.

Depending on the size and nature of the school, these emergency materials may be housed in a portable box similar to a large fishing tackle box or in a metal tool box on rollers. A larger cart can house bulky items such as emergency suctioning equipment. Regardless of size, the box should be capable of being locked, but accessed quickly. Small, breakable plastic locks can assist in safe-guarding the contents without hindering adult entry.

The actual contents of emergency carts may vary somewhat, based on the anticipated needs of the children and the staffing available. Table 9-1 lists injectable, oral and topic medications, dressing materials, and equipment and instruments appropriate in a setting employing a nurse. Modifications in the types of medication and equipment may be required if no nurse is available in your setting.

To facilitate emergency responses, it is helpful to adhere a chart summarizing complete directions for cardiopulmonary resuscitation, emergency choking responses, and poison control numbers to the top of the emergency cart. This does not preclude training and certification in these procedures, but does provide a backup.

Emergency carts should be located out of the reach of children, yet in highly visible and easily accessible areas. It is important to make two observations. First, avoid locking emergency carts in a

TABLE 9-1. Emergency Cart Inventory.

Oral Medications
Benadryl Syrup
Ipecac Syrup (to be given with warm water); check with Poison Control
Center before giving. Replace yearly to assure potency. Poison
Control number: 1-800-282-3171
Tylenol or similar liquid
Measuring spoons for measuring medication
Disposable spoons for medication administration
Physician orders for emergency medication administration, updated
yearly

Topical Medications
Ammonia inhalants
Antibacterial ointment
Hydrogen peroxide
Eye wash
Betadine Solution
Applicator sticks
Physician orders for emergency medication administration, updated
yearly

Dressings and Supplies
Packaged hand cleanser or alcohol wipes
Cotton balls for cleansing
Soap for cleansing
Dressings, varied sizes—sterile
Eye pads
Band-Aid type bandages
Ace bandage
Triangular bandage—sling
Burn sheets
Gauze bandage
Nonirritating tape (various types and sizes)—Dermiclear
Sterile gloves
Bandage scissors

Equipment and Instruments
Breakable plastic cart locks
Cold pack for sprains and bruises
Magnifying glass, needles, and tweezers for removing foreign objects
Thermometers (rectal and oral)
Thermometer sheaths
Thermometer disinfectant
Blood pressure manometer and cuffs (for infant, child, and adult)
Stethoscope (with heads for child and adult)
Penlight

(continued)

TABLE 9-1. *(continued)*

Tongue blades

Splinter forceps

Suction machine and various sizes of tubing for infants and young children (including 8, 10, and 14 French), if indicated by the needs of the children in your care; attach directions for use of the suction machine

Emergency airways for child and adults

Emergency oxygen tank and tubing, if indicated by the needs of children in your care (include emergency doctor's orders for rates)

Emergency electrical generator, if indicated by the needs of children in your center (and directions)

Disposable, nonsterile gloves

Blanket

Cleanser for cleaning equipment

Clorox or similar liquid for making 1:10 chlorine solution for cleaning blood spills

Ambu bag (with neonate, infant, child, and adult masks); attached written guidelines for rates

Regular size flashlight and current batteries

Mouth-to-mask resuscitator (child and adult)

Cervical collar

Paper cups

Hot water bottle

Safety pins

Splints

closet or office. All too often, the occupant has gone to lunch and no one has the keys to the office housing the emergency equipment. Second, do not be reluctant to place emergency carts in areas that parents may see, for fear of alarming the parents. If parents are oriented to the presence of the carts as part of the school's enrollment orientation to emergency carts and procedures, they will not be frightened. Instead, most parents will appreciate the extra precautions the school is taking to safeguard their child.

STAFF TRAINING

One of the most critical parts of emergency preparation is adequate and appropriate professional and support personnel. This group includes all interdisciplinary personnel working directly with children, as well as secretarial and related support staff working in the immediate area.

Staff training should include prevention of emergencies, as well as appropriate actions to take in an emergency. Preparation should include training and certification in basic first aid, including management of emergency illness or accident. (Readers are referred to their local American Red Cross for information about first aid courses.) Additionally, personnel should be certified in pediatric cardiopulmonary resuscitation. (Readers are referred to the local chapter of the American Heart Association for information about local courses in pediatric cardiopulmonary resuscitation. In addition, many hospitals offer community service programs in the areas at no cost or for a nominal fee.)

Emergency training should also include information about the center's emergency plan; location of emergency phones and telephone numbers; location of emergency cards; location of emergency carts; contents and use of carts; evacuation information and procedures; and special considerations in dealing with the needs of individual children and their unique situations. Unannounced evacuation drills should take place regularly and at different times of the school day. Arrangements should be made to move the children to another predetermined location, if indicated.

LIFE-THREATENING EMERGENCIES: WHAT TO DO FIRST

There are some situations that require immediate, appropriate responses within minutes. **Emergency responses must be instituted by the nearest available adult.** Do not take time to find the school nurse, even if there is one in your school. You will not have time to contact medical or emergency personnel or to take the child to the nearest hospital. Every member of the school's professional and support staff must be capable of identifying a life-threatening situation and providing emergency assistance.

An emergency situation is scary. This is especially true if it is unexpected. The first thing to do is to stay calm. Stay with the child. If another adult is available, the second person can call for necessary assistance. Prior training in first aid and cardiopulmonary resuscitation, with frequent reviews, will help give you the confidence that you need. Remember, your calm manner will help you and others around you.

The next step is to determine if the situation is life-threatening. Be sure the child's airway is open, breathing is normal, the heart is working, and bleeding is controlled. If these conditions do not exist, institute emergency resuscitation measures. (Detailed directions are in the following section.)

If a second person is available, have that person call the local emergency medical services team and bring the emergency cart to you. Start emergency first aid. If a third person is available, have that person bring the emergency cart to you while the second person is calling for emergency assistance.

The third person can then pull the Emergency Contact Card. The parent should be contacted, the situation explained, and arrangements made for the parent to meet the school representative at the school or hospital. It is imperative that the school representative remains very calm and does not alarm the parent unduly. Parents are easily alarmed with a telephone call from the school, even if it is not an emergency. Explain that school staff are trained in emergency resuscitation and first aid, and that these efforts have been started. Inform the parent if the emergency medical services team has been notified. Ascertain whether the parent seems too upset to drive to the school. If so, suggest alternative methods of transportation (i.e., a ride with a nearby friend or relative).

If the parent lacks immediate transportation, provide assurance that a school representative will remain with the child until the parent arrives. Make arrangements to meet at the hospital. The parent's presence and signature may be required by the hospital for certain kinds of treatment.

Also, attempt to contact the child's personal physician. The physician will probably want to share patient medical information with the emergency medical services team and the hospital. The physician will also need to be aware of any emergency treatment, so appropriate changes in medications and treatments can be instituted.

RESPONSES TO COMMON LIFE-THREATENING EMERGENCIES

The following sections, although not an inclusive list, will provide guidance in the identification and management of life-threatening situations.

Airway Obstruction (Choking)

This is one of the most common emergencies in infants and toddlers and a leading cause of death. Children with special health problems are often more at risk. In many cases, airway obstruction is related directly to choking. Several factors may contribute to choking episodes: (1) decreased gag reflex; (2) incomplete chewing; (3) large bites of food; (4) certain types of medications; (5) missing teeth; and (6) lack of awareness of danger (Orelove & Sobsey, 1987). Avoidance of potentially dangerous foods such as peanuts, marshmallows, grapes, hot dogs, and hard candies can help reduce deaths from choking (Holvoet & Helmstetter, 1989). Selection of appropriate food consistency and texture, and appropriate positioning during feeding will also help to reduce the incidence of choking episodes.

In some situations, a foreign object obstructs the airway. Removal of balloons and small toys from play areas used by infants and toddlers will eliminate many risks. Fuzzy toys, small objects, and pieces of lint should be removed from the environment of a child with a tracheostomy. This precaution will reduce the potential for the child to place the item directly into the tracheostomy opening. Careful observation and postural drainage or suctioning of mucus accumulations is needed for many children with respiratory illness.

Early symptoms may be very subtle. They may include restlessness and irritability, and increased respiratory rate and pulse. If the child can still cry or talk, the obstruction is not complete. Give the child an opportunity to clear the obstruction without external assistance. Indeed, maneuvers may even prove to dangerous (American Academy of Pediatrics, 1988). Be sure to carefully observe the child to determine if the condition improves, or if it worsens and emergency response is indicated.

During the first few minutes after obstruction, the symptoms become more noticeable. The child may be very irritated or abnormally quiet. The child may have a very weak or ineffective cough, cry silently, or clutch at the throat. Within minutes, the skin will become deep red or purple. As the child becomes less oxygenated, the skin will gradually turn blue or gray. The child will lose consciousness and attempt to breath less frequently. Death will occur within 5 minutes if the obstruction is not removed.

Attempts to clear the airway should be considered when: (a) you have observed the aspiration or strongly suspect it; (b) the child is unconscious and nonbreathing, and whose airway remains apparently obstructed despite usual methods of clearing (American Medical Association, 1986).

As soon as you notice that the infant or child is not breathing normally, begin the following interventions:

1. Remain calm and reassure the victim.
2. Determine if the victim is unconscious. Try to elicit a response by gently shaking the victim and shouting "Are you ok?" If the child can cry or speak, do not interfere with the child's own attempts to clear the airway. If the child may have had head or neck injuries, take special care to avoid damaging the spinal cord.

3. If there is no response, call out for help and proceed to attempt to open the airway. If you are alone, perform CPR for 1 minute before going for help.

These three points are used for any infant or child. From this point, interventions may vary depending on the following specific situations.

If an infant (under 1 year of age) is conscious, (do not use the Heimlich Maneuver for this age group) do the following:

1. Position the infant prone over the rescuer's forearm, with the infant's legs straddling the forearm. The infant's head should be down, jaw firmly supported, and positioned lower than the trunk. The rescuer's forearm should rest on his or her thigh for additional support.
2. Deliver four back blows to the area between the infant's shoulder blades, using the heel of the rescuer's hand (Figure 9-2).
3. If the obstruction is not relieved, support the infant's head, neck, and chest with one hand and the infant's back with the other and turn the infant over as one unit.

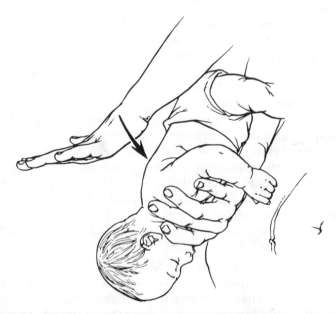

Figure 9-2. Positioning an infant for back blows. *Textbook of pediatric advanced life support,* 1988. Copyright American Heart Association. Reproduced with permission.

4. Place the infant on his or her back, with the head down. Be sure to support the head and neck.
5. Using two to three fingers, apply four chest thrusts. Depress the sternum 1/2 to 1 inch with each thrust. **Due to risk of injury to vital organs in the abdomen, do not use abdominal thrusts in infants under one year of age (Figure 9-3).**
6. If breathing is not resumed, check again for a foreign body. Manually remove it if present. If no foreign body is noted, attempt ventilation with two breaths by mouth-to-mouth or mouth-to-nose technique. Repeat back blows and chest thrusts until the foreign body is expelled, while seeking aid from emergency medical services.

If the infant is unconscious for no obvious reason, do the following:

1. Place the infant on his or her back on a firm, hard surface. Keep the infant's face up. Place your thumb in the infant's mouth, over the tongue. Attempt to open the airway using the head-tilt, chin-lift method (Figure 9-4).
2. Check the infant's mouth for the presence of the foreign object.
3. Remove the foreign object only if it is seen.

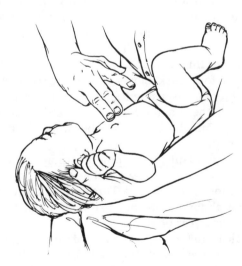

Figure 9-3. Positioning an infant for chest thrusts. *Textbook of pediatric advanced life support*, 1988. Copyright American Heart Association. Reproduced with permission.

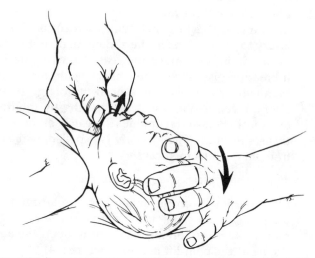

Figure 9-4. Head tilt, chin lift. *Textbook of pediatric advanced life support*, 1988. Copyright American Heart Association. Reproduced with permission.

4. Attempt to ventilate. Seal the infant's mouth and nose with your mouth, and attempt to breathe into the infant's mouth.
5. If the airway is obstructed, position the infant prone over the rescuer's forearm, with the infant's head down and the jaw firmly supported. The rescuer's forearm then rests on his or her thigh.
6. Deliver four back blows to the area between the infant's shoulder blades, using the heel of the rescuer's hand.
7. Support the infant's head, neck, and chest with one hand and the infant's back with the other. Turn the infant over as one unit.
8. Place the infant in a supine position, with head down. Be sure to support the head and neck.
9. Apply four chest thrusts. **Due to risk of injury to vital organs in the abdomen, do not use abdominal thrusts in infants under one year of age.**
10. Check again for a foreign body. Manually remove it if present, using tongue-jaw lift (Figure 9-5).
11. If the foreign body is removed, and the victim is not breathing, repeat the steps to open the airway, perform rescue breathing, and do chest compressions.

12. If the foreign body is not removed, continue the sequence: attempt rescue breathing, and do back blows and chest thrusts. Attempt to see the object.

For a conscious child over 1 year of age, standing or sitting, use the Heimlich Maneuver (subdiaphragmatic abdominal thrusts).

1. Position the child in front of the rescuer.
2. Position the rescuer's arms around the child and grasp in front of the child's waist, with one hand made into a fist.
3. Place the rescuer's fist on the child's waist, above the navel and below the sternum (Figure 9-6).
4. Grasp the fist with the other hand and apply a quick, upward thrust against victim's abdomen.
5. Check the mouth for dislodged foreign materials. Repeat abdominal thrust six to eight times, if necessary.

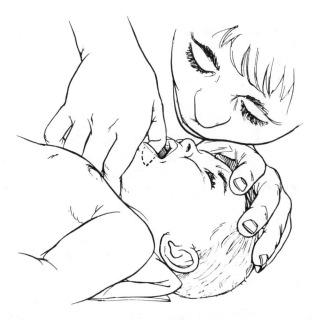

Figure 9-5. Tongue-jaw lift. *Textbook of pediatric advanced life support,* 1988. Copyright American Heart Association. Reproduced with permission.

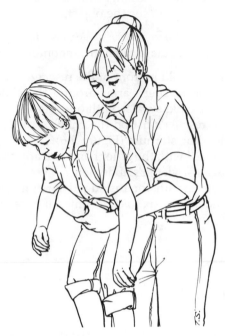

Figure 9-6. Heimlich maneuver: Child standing or sitting (conscious). *Textbook of pediatric advanced life support*, 1988. Copyright American Heart Association. Reproduced with permission.

For an unconscious child over 1 year of age, use the Heimlich Maneuver (subdiaphragmatic abdominal thrusts).

1. Use the tongue/jaw lift to open the mouth and look for the foreign object.
2. If no foreign object is visible, use the head tilt/child lift to position the airway and attempt rescue breathing. If it is unsuccessful, begin the Heimlich Maneuver.
3. Position the child on its back, with the rescuer kneeling at the child's feet.
4. Place the heel of one of the rescuer's hands in the middle of the child's abdomen, above the navel and below the sternum.
5. Place the rescuer's second hand over the fist and press into the child's abdomen, using a quick, upward thrust.
6. Check the mouth for dislodged foreign materials using the tongue/jaw lift. No blind finger sweeps should be used. If the object is seen, remove it. If an object is not seen, attempt

to ventilate the child. If unsuccessful, repeat the abdominal thrust six to eight times (Figure 9-7). Continue the sequence until successful, or emergency assistance arrives.

Airway Obstruction in a Child with a Tracheostomy: Emergency Tube Replacement

Sometimes a child with a tracheostomy suffers from an airway obstruction. This problem can occur if the tracheostomy is accidentally removed or pulled out by the child. An obstruction can also occur if foreign material (such as a toy) blocks the tracheostomy tube itself, or if suctioning is not effective in removing mucous from the tracheostomy tube.

If these situations occur, emergency tube replacement may be necessary. Selected child care workers should be specially trained in this technique prior to the child's first day at school with a tracheostomy. Training should include return demonstrations and periodic supervision by a physician or nurse. (Table 9-2 details the emergency tube replacement procedure.)

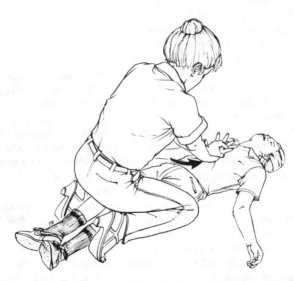

Figure 9-7. Heimlich maneuver: Child lying (unconscious). *Textbook of pediatric advanced life support*, 1988. Copyright American Heart Association. Reproduced with permission.

TABLE 9-2. Emergency Tube Replacement.

Perform this procedure if you are unable to provide an open airway after 3 suctioning attempts; if the child exhibits signs of extreme difficulty in breathing; or if the tracheostomy tube has been accidentally removed. IT IS RECOMMENDED THAT TWO TRAINED ADULTS BE PRESENT DURING THIS PROCEDURE.

Equipment

1. Stand-by tracheostomy tube, of the type and size prescribed by the child's physician. Be sure to have an obturator if one is needed for the prescribed tracheostomy tube. The tracheostomy tube will be clean or sterile, depending on physician's orders. (Extra tubes should be on hand at all times.)
2. Sterile tracheostomy tube of next smaller size. (Extra tube should be on hand at all times.)
3. Bandage scissors
4. Small blanket roll (optional in emergency)
5. Tracheostomy ties (twill tape or velcro band)
6. Sterile saline
7. Manual resuscitator (Ambu bag) with tracheostomy adapter
8. Oxygen source, if ordered by the child's physician
9. Gloves (sterile or clean, as ordered by the child's physician).

Procedure

1. Comfort and reassure the child and explain the procedure, as time permits
2. Gather equipment
3. Wash hands, if time permits
4. If possible, place the child on the back, with a small blanket roll under the neck. This will enable you to see the tracheostomy opening (stoma) more easily. Omit this step, if necessary.
5. If the old tracheostomy tube is in place, follow routine tracheostomy tube changing procedure. (Refer to Chapter 6, if time permits.)
6. If the old tracheostomy tube is not in the stoma, pick up the new tracheostomy tube by the flanges (wings). Do not touch the tube itself. Apply a small amount of sterile saline to the longest end of the new tracheostomy tube. (Moistening of the new tracheostomy tube facilitates insertion.)
7. Hold the new tracheostomy tube in your dominant hand. If necessary, spread the child's stoma open with the index and middle finger of your other hand.
8. Put the new tracheostomy tube into the stoma. Direct the tube at right angle and rotate downward to correct position; insertion can be facilitated by pulling tube back 1/4 inch, then easing it in by turning slightly side to side. Remove the obturator which

(continued)

TABLE 9-2.   *(continued)*

occludes the tracheostomy tube. (*Note:* some types of tracheostomy tubes do not have an obturator to guide insertion.)

9. If the trachea starts to spasm as you are inserting the new tube, apply pressure with the new tracheostomy tube until the stoma opens.

10. Listen, to be sure air is being exchanged through the new tube. Keep a manual resuscitator and oxygen ready. If the child is not breathing, give artificial respiration by mouth-to-stoma breathing or via manual resuscitator.

11. Hold the tube in place until a second person can place new ties on the tracheostomy phlenges. (Refer to routine tracheostomy changes in Chapter 6, if time permits. Remember to keep the ties loose enough to permit one finger to be inserted between the knot and the child's neck.

12. Suction, if necessary. (Refer to Chapter 6, if time permits.)

13. *If you are unable to insert the new tracheostomy tube due to tube not fitting into stoma or stoma closing:*

    a. Reposition the child's neck and try again
    b. If a new tracheostomy tube will not enter, try to insert the tracheostomy tube in the next smaller size.
    c. If the smaller tube will not enter, place a suction catheter in the stoma, and cut it off about 6 inches from the stoma. *Do not let go of the catheter. Call for emergency assistance.* Prepare to transfer the child when help arrives.

14. Observe the child to be sure breathing is easier.

15. Wash hands.

16. Notify parent and physician.

17. Document procedure. Include date, time, reason for action and child's response.

Adapted from Urbano, M. T. (1989). *Children's medical services nursing procedure reference guide.* Tallahassee, FL: Florida Department of Health and Rehabilitative Services, with permission.

If any of the following situations occur, the emergency medical services team should be called immediately.

Severe Breathing Difficulties

Some children may have serious breathing difficulties but may not have an actual airway obstruction. Difficulty with breathing may be caused by the child's condition itself (i.e., asthma, Sudden Infant Death syndrome, or a severe respiratory tract infection); a severe allergic reaction; drowning; suffocation caused by foreign objects such as toys, foods, or plastic; smoke inhalation; injury, or electrical shock.

Early symptoms include restlessness, irritability, and increased respiratory and pulse rates. Later symptoms include noisy or weak or nonexistent breathing; possible loss of consciousness; enlarged pupils; and bluish color of lips, tongue, and fingernail beds (*Note:* In a black person, these may appear chalky gray).

Responses to severe breathing difficulties should include the following sequence:

1. Determine if the child is breathing. Position the child on a firm, flat surface. However, if there is possibility of head or neck injury, do not move the child unless it is critically necessary.

2. Position the child's airway open. This action can be accomplished when the head is straightened and the jaw is lifted. Take precautions. If there is evidence of an injury to the head or neck, use the jaw-thrust maneuver to open the airway (see Figure 9-8).

3. Assess breathing by looking for chest movement, placing your ear over the child's mouth and listening for exhaled air and feeling for exhaled air (see Figure 9-9).

4. If the child is not breathing, begin *rescue breathing.*

   a. Take a breath, yourself.

   b. Place your mouth over the nose and mouth of the child. (For an older child, put your mouth over the child's mouth and occlude the child's nose by pinching the child's nostrils with your fingers).

   c. Force breath into the victim's mouth. Use just enough pressure to cause the child's chest to rise. In infants, it is best to use puffs of air. Allow the chest to deflate, then breathe again. If the rescuer's breath is not enough to raise the chest wall, try slightly stronger breaths. *Note:*

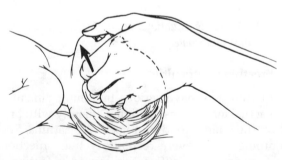

Figure 9-8. Jaw-thrust. *Textbook of pediatric advanced life support*, 1988. Copyright American Heart Association. Reproduced with permission.

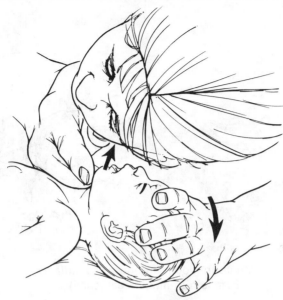

Figure 9-9. Assessment: Determining breathlessness while maintaining head tilt/chin lift—look, listen, feel. *Textbook of pediatric advanced life support*, 1988. Copyright American Heart Association. Reproduced with permission.

Inability to inflate the lungs confirms a blocked airway.(Holvoet & Helmstetter, 1989). *Responses for an airway obstruction should be instituted immediately* (Figure 9-10).

d. After two initial breaths, feel the brachial pulse in an infant. It is on the inner side of the upper arm midway between the elbow and the shoulder (Figure 9-11). In an older child, feel the neck for the carotid pulse (Figure 9-12). If a pulse is present, continue rescue breathing only (Infant: 20 times per minute; Child: 15 times per minute.) Continue until spontaneous breathing occurs.

e. If no pulse is present, initiate cardiac resuscitation. (Refer to Heart Stoppage section following.)

f. *Note:* Rescue breathing can contribute to abdominal distention and/or vomiting if the rescuer breathes too large a volume of air into the child, if the rescue breathing is too rapid or if the airway is not completely open. If the child vomits, turn the head and body to the side to prevent choking, clean out the mouth, and resume rescue breathing, as indicated.

g. *Note:* Have the child evaluated by a physician, even if breathing has resumed.

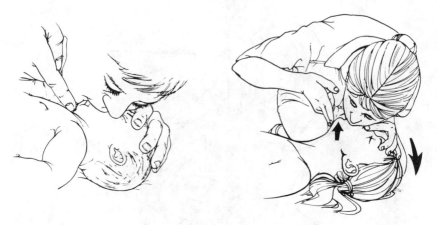

A. Mouth-to-mouth-and-nose seal (infant)
B: mouth-to-mouth-seal (child)

Figure 9-10. Breathing for the victim. *Textbook of pediatric advanced life support,* 1988. Copyright American Heart Association. Reproduced with permission.

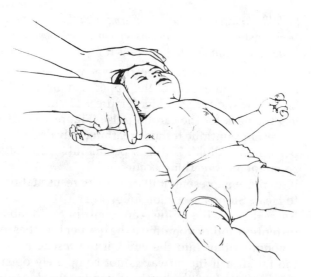

Figure 9-11. Palpating the brachial pulse (infant). *Textbook of pediatric advanced life support,* 1988. Copyright American Heart Association. Reproduced with permission.

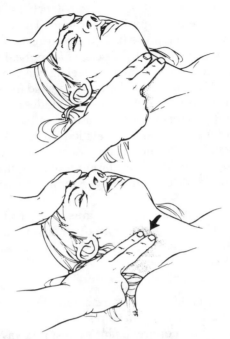

Figure 9-12. Palpating the carotid pulse (child). *Textbook of pediatric advanced life support,* 1988. Copyright American Heart Association. Reproduced with permission.

Severe Breathing Difficulties in a Child with a Tracheostomy

If a child with a tracheostomy appears to be having difficulty breathing, suctioning may help to clear the airway. (Refer to Chapter 6 for further discussions about tracheostomies and their care.)

If the child is still having difficulty breathing, mouth to stoma (tracheostomy opening) resuscitation may be indicated. This is basically the same technique as rescue breathing, except that the rescuer's mouth is over the tracheostomy opening. An appropriately sized manual resuscitator (ambu bag) may also be used. An ambu bag is essentially an air-filled bellows with a mask. The rescuer alternately compresses and releases the ambu bag which in turn delivers air to the victim via the tracheostomy adaptor. The overall procedure and rates are similar to those for mouth-to-mouth resuscitation.

Heart Stoppage

Heart stoppage (cardiac arrest) is not as common in infants and children as it is in adults. More commonly, heart stoppage occurs from a circulatory or respiratory problem (such as obstruction of the airway or extreme difficulty in breathing). These situations can precipitate cessation of the pulse (i.e., cardiac arrest).

Heart stoppage is indicated by absence of a pulse. Presence or absence of a pulse can be determined by feeling the brachial artery in an infant (Figure 9-11) or the carotid artery in a child (Figure 9-12).

The correct response to heart stoppage includes cardiopulmonary resuscitation (CPR). In this technique, attempts to open the airway and restore breathing are made, as detailed previously. In addition, external compression of the chest is necessary to get the heart pumping again. Cardiopulmonary resuscitation must begin within 4 minutes after the pulse and breathing have stopped to save the child's life.

If the child is not breathing, you must be sure that the heart has not stopped. While maintaining an open airway, simultaneously feel for a pulse. If it can not be felt after 5 to 10 seconds, it indicates that circulation is compromised.

For an infant, do the following:

1. Position the child on a flat surface, and begin chest compressions, in addition to artificial respiration.
2. Locate a position on the infant's chest midway between the child's nipples; position the rescuer's index finger one fingerbreadth below that point (Figure 9-13).

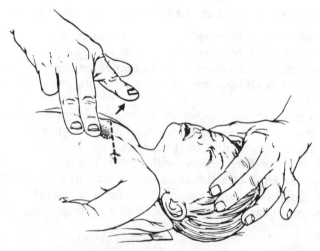

Figure 9-13. Locating the correct position for the fingers in chest compressions in the infant. *Textbook of pediatric advanced life support,* 1988. Copyright American Heart Association. Reproduced with permission.

3. Using two fingers, compress the breastbone (sternum) to a depth of 1/2 to 1 inch.

4. Release pressure without moving the fingers from that location.

5. Repeat 100 times per minute. (Intersperse one breath after each 5 compressions.)

6. Feel for a pulse. If it is present, stop cardiac compressions. If there is no pulse, continue CPR.

For a child, do the following:

1. Locate a position on the child's chest, at the place where the child's rib cage meets the base of the breastbone (sternum) (Figure 9-14).

2. Put the rescuer's middle finger on that location, and the index finger next to it. Place the heel of the hand next to the index finger.

3. Use one hand to compress the chest 1 to 1½ inches.

4. Repeat 80 to 100 times per minute. Intersperse one breath after each 5 compressions.

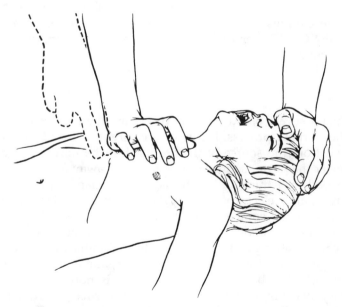

Figure 9-14. Locating the correct position for the hand in chest compressions in the child. *Textbook of pediatric advanced life support,* 1988. Copyright American Heart Association. Reproduced with permission.

5. Feel for a pulse. If it is present, stop cardiac compressions. If there is no pulse, continue CPR.

Note: If the rescuer is alone and finds a child who is not breathing or has no pulse, or both, start CPR. If the breathing or pulse have not started again after 1 minute, telephone for help and return immediately to the child to reinstitute CPR. Once CPR has been restarted, it should be continued until the child's heart starts beating, an emergency medical services team takes over, or the rescuer is too tired to continue.

Severe or Extensive Burns

There are three levels of burns: first, second and third degree. When there are first degree burns, the skin is red (like a sunburn) but there are no blisters or white patches. This burn is uncomfortable, but it will heal in a few days.

Second degree burns are red with either blisters or white patches. This burn is worse than a first degree burn. If the area is small, keep cold water on the burn for several hours. If it is a large area, the child should be seen by a doctor.

Third degree burns are the worst. In this type of burn, a whole layer of skin has been damaged or destroyed. It may not hurt, because the nerve endings have been destroyed. This type of burn is an **EMERGENCY**. The emergency medical services team should be called immediately.

First Aid

When a severe or extensive burn occurs, the rescuer must first stop the burning process. In the case of fire, this entails removing the child from the source of the fire itself. If the burn is electrical, disconnect the power source, or pull the child away from the source using wood or a thick, dry cloth, never bare hands. Failure to do this may result in electrical burns to the rescuer. Following the child's removal from the source of the burn, the child should be placed in a horizontal position if possible. Check for an open airway and presence of breathing and a pulse. As indicated, initiate CPR. Summon the emergency medical services system team, and notify the parent.

If the child is breathing and the pulse is normal, CPR is not necessary. Begin other emergency procedures while you wait for the emergency medical services system team to arrive.

Allow for spontaneous cooling of the burned area by putting the area in cold water or applying cool wet compresses to the injured area. This is particularly important if there is a chemical burn. However, do not apply water if the chemical is a powder. The addition of water will result in further spread of the caustic materials. Do not apply ice water or ice packs to the burned area. These will just cause further damage.

Whenever possible, remove the burned clothing. This will stop further burning and avoid painful removal later. Cover the burned area with a clean cloth to prevent contamination and reduce pain due to exposure of the burned areas to air. Do not apply any ointments or other treatments. Do not give anything by mouth.

Regardless of the size of the burn, a physician should be consulted anytime a burn breaks the skin or an electrical burn occurs. A physician should also be consulted immediately anytime there is a burn on the face, hands, feet, or genitalia (American Academy of Pediatrics, 1987).

For serious, deep burns, call for an emergency medical services team. Do *not* apply cold water or any medication. Cover the child with a clean cloth, and then a blanket.

Severe Bleeding

Remember to use gloves whenever you come in contact with blood or objects contaminated by blood. This precaution will prevent the possible spread of infection to both you and the victim. (Refer to Chapter 8 for further information on Universal Precautions.)

First Aid

Many wounds, especially head wounds, cause large amounts of bleeding. Regardless of the degree of injury, measures to control bleeding should be taken immediately. Bleeding can be stopped by applying direct pressure to the wound or pressure at the pulse points.

Gross debris can be removed from the wound, but not if a large object is penetrating the child. If a large penetrating object is present, cover the wound with a clean or sterile dressing, and apply direct pressure over the wound, or at pressure points. (Refer to a standard first aid book if you need a review of pressure points.) Medical evaluation of the child should be obtained in all cases of internal or extensive bleeding.

Severed Body Part

If the bleeding is due to a severed body part, control the bleeding first. Wet sterile or clean gauze in water or sterile saline, if it is available.

Place this damp gauze over the stump. Put some waterproof covering over the stump, then wrap in an ice-filled plastic bag. Also wrap the severed body part with gauze and place it in an ice-filled container. (Avoid direct contact between the ice and the skin.) Label the container with the child's name, date, and time. Have the emergency medical services team transport the child to the emergency room as soon as possible. Be sure to take the severed body part to the hospital with the child. Many times, the surgeon can reattach the severed part.

Internal Bleeding

Signs of faintness, rapid pulse rate, thirst, and cold sweaty skin may indicate internal bleeding. Get medical advise immediately.

Injuries

It is especially important to provide immediate first aid to injuries of the head, neck, back, chest, abdomen, or eye.

Head

Head injuries always have the potential for being dangerous. Be sure to observe the child for loss of consciousness. Persistent unconsciousness may indicate internal injury and must be immediately evaluated by a physician.

Initial first aid involves being sure the airway is clear and open, the heart is still beating, and bleeding is controlled. If not, open the airway, and initiate rescue breathing or CPR, as indicated.

Next, determine the cause and extent of the injury. Have the child evaluated immediately by a physician if: the injury was the result of great force (high speed, fall from a great distance); the victim is an infant (under 6 months of age); was unconscious for more than 5 seconds; demonstrates headache, dizziness or pale color lasting longer than one hour after injury; persistent vomiting (3 or more times); unequal, dilated or fixed pupils; unusual behavior or difficulty in being aroused; there is any oozing of blood or watery fluid from the ears or nose; swelling in front or above ear; or if the child develops paralysis or difficulty in moving an arm or leg, or maintaining balance.

Even if the child does not demonstrate these symptoms immediately after the injury, complete rest should follow the incident. Be sure to notify the parent of any injury. Instruct them to carefully observe the child for the next 24 to 48 hours, to assure possible complications will be detected early.

Neck or Back

Injury to the neck or spinal cord may be apparent by swelling, bruising, penetrating wounds, or deformity of the area due to the injury. Spinal cord injury is also suspected if the child loses feeling or motor ability. If injury to the neck or spinal cord is even vaguely suspected, keep the child still and quiet. Avoid moving the child unless there is immediate danger. Wait until the emergency medical services team arrives and takes proper precautions prior to moving the child.

Chest Injuries

Injuries of the chest may indicate serious underlying damage to vital organs. Especially if the injury is penetrating or crushing, the child should be closely observed for signs of bleeding or difficulty breathing. The child should receive prompt medical evaluation.

Abdomen

Observe for signs of swelling, bruising, penetrating wounds, or bleeding at the urinary meatus (external opening to the urinary tract) or the genitalia. Such injury can indicate serious damage to internal organs.

Eye Injuries

Eyes can be injured by blows, cuts, penetrating objects, or burns from heat and corrosive substances. All eye injuries should be treated very seriously. Do not permit the eye to be rubbed, and do not use any eye medication.

If the injury has been caused by a penetrating object, do not attempt to irrigate (wash out) the eye or remove the object. If the injury is due to a chemical burn, hold the lids open and irrigate the eye copiously with tap water for 20 minutes. A gentle continuous stream of water from a pitcher works well. Any eye injury, especially if it is penetrating or corrosive should be immediately evaluated by a physician.

Accidental Poisoning

Infants, toddlers, and preschoolers are at special risk for accidental poisoning. Developmentally, they are exploring their environments, and everything seems to end up in their mouths. Ingestion of a variety of materials including some plants, cleaning substances, cosmetics, medications, and alcohol may poison the child. Preventative measures to keep poisons out of the reach of children are critical.

Suspect poisoning if the actual ingestion was observed; if an open, spilled or empty container is found and the child could have ingested the contents; if there is odor of poison on the child's breath or clothes; or if the child is found unconscious in conjunction with any of the previous conditions.

If these situations occur, observe respirations and pulse. Initiate cardiopulmonary resuscitation as necessary.

If the child's lungs and heart seem to be working properly, take the child and the poison container to the phone, and call the Poison Control number. (It should be listed on the top of your emergency cart.)

Do not follow the directions for responding to accident poisoning that may be on the label of a container. These directions may not be accurate for the size or age of the child in your care.

Give Syrup of Ipecac from the Emergency Cart only if the Poison Control staff tell you to administer it. Be sure to tell the Poison Control Center if the child is likely to have difficulty vomiting, is at increased risk for aspirating if vomiting occurs, of if any abnormalities of the esophagus, throat or stomach already exist.

The Syrup of Ipecac will induce vomiting. Give only the amount of water the Poison Control staff tell you. Large amounts of water may enhance gastric emptying, thereby forcing the poison further into the digestive tract.

Induction of vomiting requires caution and good judgment. Vomiting of some materials such as strong corrosives (such as drain cleaner), or petroleum products (such as furniture polish and gasoline) can cause further damage. Do not attempt to neutralize corrosives by giving vinegar or lemon juice, unless instructed by the Poison Center. The resulting thermal chemical reaction can result in additional burning. Do not induce vomiting if the child is unconscious or drowsy, or demonstrating uncontrolled body movements unless you are told to by the Poison Control Center. These symptoms may indicate central nervous system depression.

Next, call the emergency medical services team and have the child taken to the hospital emergency room for medical evaluation. Be sure to send any vomited materials, the package or container which contained the suspected poison, and whatever was left of the suspected material.

Continuous Seizures (Status Epilepticus)

Seizures are common in infants, toddlers, and preschoolers with developmental delays and disabilities. Some of these seizures are so severe that they are not controlled by medication, or even by a combination of very powerful medications. Consequently, seizure activity in a child with a history of failure to control similar seizures may not, in itself, be an emergency situation. (Refer to Chapter 6 for complete discussion of seizures.) However, seizure activity in a child who has not had previous seizures is in need of medical evaluation.

Status Epilepticus

Although rare, a child may have continuous seizures called **status epilepticus, which is a medical emergency.** Status epilepticus is a state of prolonged seizure or a series of seizures during which the child does not resume consciousness. This condition most frequently occurs in a child with epilepsy when medication has been changed or is not being taken as prescribed, when the child's anticonvulsant medication has been stopped suddenly, or when the child's body has been stressed by an additional illness. If a child does not have epilepsy, it may be the result of a severe head injury.

A single seizure or continuous series of seizures lasting a total of 10 minutes is considered to be an indication of possible status epilepticus. Thus, if any seizure occurs, the starting time should be noted for future information. If nursing support is available in your setting, notify the nurse of any seizure lasting 3 minutes or more, so the nurse can assist in emergency management.

For seizures lasting more than 5 minutes, request emergency assistance from the emergency medical services team. If the team takes the child to the hospital, be sure to send along a list of the child's medications, completed seizure logs, and the time of last medication administration (if known). Lack of prompt treatment may result in brain damage and death. However, with quick treatment, the child may be able to survive without long-term damage.

WHEN THE EMERGENCY MEDICAL SERVICES TEAM ARRIVES

Continue giving emergency first aid until the emergency medical services team arrives. If possible, have someone posted by the road to direct the rescue team to the exact location of the child. When the team arrives, give them a brief summary of the child's age and diagnosis, description of the emergency, the child's response, and emergency actions taken. Then move out of the way, so the team can work.

Have someone else gather the child's emergency card, a description of the child's health needs and routine medications, and the permission form for emergency treatment. If the parent is not present, have one adult go with the emergency team to the hospital.That adult should be someone who knows what happened, and, ideally, someone who has a good relationship with the family. Be sure the other children in the setting have adequate supervision.

AFTER THE EMERGENCY

You have handled yourself and the situation well. With the child safely in the care of the emergency team, the parent or the hospital, it is now time to gather loose ends.

First, let all the other staff and the children in the class know that the ill or injured child is safe and is receiving good care. Even young and involved children can sense that something has happened and need to be reassured.

Then, turn to paperwork. No school-based emergency is really complete until recording is finished. Each school should have a specific form to record incidents of serious accidents or illness. (Figure 9-15 presents a sample.) Such a form should be completed whenever an accident occurs, a child is injured, or illness is severe enough to disrupt the child's participation in school activities. Note the emergency and the medical interventions the child received, as well as any prescribed medication or activity restrictions. You may need to wait until you contact the physician to obtain this information. Accurate and comprehensive completion is essential because this paperwork provides legal documentation of the event. Give one copy to the parent, and retain one for the file.

NON LIFE-THREATENING EMERGENCIES

Fortunately, most emergencies are not life-threatening. In these situations, basic responses are similar. First, determine that the child is not having difficulty with breathing, circulation or bleeding. Next, be sure other life-saving responses are not indicated. Following those basic steps, routine first aid can be administered.

Responses following the administration of first aid depend on the status of the child. If the situation is relatively minor, the child may remain in school. However, the child should remain under observation to be sure no complications arise. If the situation is more severe, but does not require an emergency medical services system team, the child probably needs to be evaluated in a clinic or in the doctor's office. In this situation, the parent should be contacted.

Again, remain very calm during your contact with the parent. Parents naturally assume the worse. You do not want to alarm the

Figure 9-15. Accident/illness report.

Child's Name: Birthdate:
Parent's Name:
Parent's Address: Parent's Phone:

Date of Accident or Illness:
Description of Accident or Illness: (Include type of accident or illness; if injury, include details).
Course of Action Taken: (Include action and person taking action)
Was the parent notified by telephone or in person? (Include date and time; parental response; action taken).
Was an Emergency Rescue Team contacted? If so, include date, time, and action taken.
Was the child's physician contacted? If so, include date, name of physician, time, action taken.
Results of Action:
Followup required: (Include any changes in medications or treatments)
Name of School Personnel Witnessing the Event:
Signature of School Personnel Witnessing the Event:
Person Completing this Report:
Date of Report:
Methods Taken to Prevent Similar Situation in the Future:

Director's Signature:
Date:

parent so much that the parent becomes involved in a traffic accident on the way to pick up the child at school.

If the situation was serious enough to contact the parent, the child should probably be moved to a quiet area for rest and further observation. The child will probably be comforted by being held and assured that the parent is on the way.

When the parent arrives, describe the emergency and the emergency actions taken. Offer to either let a school representative who was present during the emergency accompany the parent to the physician's office, or to call the physician and provide a summary of the situation. Request that the parent call after the physician's evaluation, thereby notifying the school of additional treatment. The parent can also be questioned regarding any changes in the child's medications or treatments, as well as the anticipated date of return to the school. In some cases, the school may request a physician's note prior to school re-entry. This is generally done to assure the school that the classroom is a safe environment for the child at that time.

If the parent does not have transportation, the child may need to be transported by a taxi, accompanied by a school representative. Do not drive the child yourself. Most insurance companies will not cover potential liability in this situation.

Sometimes, neither the parent nor the emergency contact is available. In this case, consult with the school nurse (if available) and/or the child's physician. Explain the situation and the child's current status. Determine if the school should arrange a medical evaluation or if it can wait until the parent can assume responsibility. If the child does not need an immediate medical evaluation, but the child should only be released in the parent's direct care, school personnel must remain with the child until the parent or other emergency contact has been located.

At other times, a potential emergency was not as serious as originally perceived. Determine if the child can be safely transported home by the usual means (bus, and so on). Contact the parent to be sure someone will be present to care for the child upon arrival home.

Always, alert the parent to signs and symptoms of complications. Instruct the parent to notify the child's physician if such symptoms occur.

SUMMARY

Emergencies are never desirable, but proper planning and training can mean the difference between incident and death. It is imperative that each interdisciplinary professional working with young children who are developmentally delayed or disabled commit to individual preparation by learning first aid and cardiopulmonary resuscitation.

BIBLIOGRAPHY

American Academy of Pediatrics. (1990). Children with health impairments in the schools. *Pediatrics, 86*(4), 636-638.

American Academy of Pediatrics. (1990). Guidelines for urgent care in the school. *Pediatrics, 86*(6), 999-1000.

American Academy of Pediatrics. (1987). *Health care in day care: A manual for health professionals.* Elk Grove, IL: Author.

American Heart Association. (1986). *First aid for choking.* Dallas, TX : Author.

Batshaw, M., & Perret, Y. (1986). *Children with handicaps: A medical primer* (2nd ed.). Baltimore: Paul H. Brookes.

Graff, J., Ault, M., Guess, D., Taylor, M., & Thompson, B. (1990). *Health care for students with disabilities.* Baltimore: Paul H. Brookes.

Newton, J. (1989). *The new school health handbook: A ready reference for school nurses and educators.* Englewood Cliffs, NJ: Prentice Hall.

Whaley, L., & Wong, D. (1987). *Nursing care for infants and children.* St. Louis: C. V. Mosby.

APPENDIX:
RESOURCE ADDRESSES

AIDS

Centers for Disease Control
404-329-3479

Public Health Service
1-800-447-AIDS

CEREBRAL PALSY

American Academy of Cerebral
Palsy and Developmental Medicine
P.O. Box 11083
Richmond, VA 23230

United Cerebral Palsy
Associations, Inc.
66 East 34th Street
New York, NY 10016

COCAINE-EXPOSED
INFANTS

Cocaine Baby Help Line
(312) 908-0867

24 Hour Toll-free information and
referral service 1-800-COCAINE

March of Dimes Birth Defects
Foundation
1275 Mamaroneck Avenue
White Plains, NY 10605

National Association for Perinatal
Addiction Research and Education
(NAPARE)
11 E. Hubbard, Suite 200
Chicago, IL 60611

National Clearinghouse for Alcohol
and Drug Information
P. O. Box 2345
Rockville, MD 20852

DOWN SYNDROME

Association for Children with Down
Syndrome
2616 Martin Avenue
Bellmore, NY 11710

March of Dimes Birth Defects
Foundation
1275 Mamaroneck Avenue
White Plains, NY 10605

National Association for Retarded
Citizens
P.O. Box 6109
Arlington, TX 76006

National Down Syndrome Congress
1800 Dempster Street
Park Ridge, IL 60068-1146

National Down Syndrome Society
666 Broadway, Suite 810
New York, NY 10012

EPILEPSY

Epilepsy Foundation of America
4351 Garden City Drive
Landover, MD 20785

HYDROCEPHALUS

Hydrocephalus Foundation of
Northern California
Box 342
2040 Polk Street
San Francisco, CA 94109

Hydrocephalus Opens Peoples Eyes
(HOPE)
104-47 120th Street
Richmond Hill, NY 11419

National Hydrocephalus Foundation
22427 S. River Road
Joliet, IL 60436

INFECTION

American Academy of Pediatrics
P.O. Box 927
141 Northwest Point Blvd
Elk Grove Village, IL 60009-0927

American Public Health Association
1015 Fifteenth Street, NW
Washington, DC 20005

Centers for Disease Control
U.S. Department of Health and
Human Services
Atlanta, GA 30333

MUSCULAR DYSTROPHY

Muscular Dystrophy Association
(MDA)
810 Seventh Avenue
New York, NY 10019

SPINA BIFIDA

Council for Exceptional Children
Division on the Physically
Handicapped
1920 Association Drive
Reston, VA 22091

March of Dimes Birth Defects
Foundation
1275 Mamaroneck Avenue
White Plains, NY 10605

National Association of the
Physically Handicapped
76 Elm Street
London, OH 43146

National Center for Education in
Child and Maternal Health
3520 Prospect Street, NW
Washington, DC 20007

National Easter Seal Society
2023 W. Ogden Avenue
Chicago, IL 60612

National Information Center for
Handicapped Children and Youth
P.O. Box 1492
Washington, DC 20013

Spina Bifida Association of America
1700 Rockville Pike
Rockville, MD 20852

REFERENCES

American Academy of Pediatrics. (1987). *Health in day care: A manual for health professionals.* Elk Grove, IL: Author.

American Academy of Pediatrics. (1988). First aid for the choking child. *Pediatrics, 81*(5), 740-742.

American Academy of Pediatrics, Task Force on Pediatric AIDS. (1988). Pediatric guidelines for infection control of Human Immunodeficiency Virus (Acquired Immunodeficiency Virus) in hospitals, medical offices, schools and other settings. *Pediatrics, 82*, 801-807.

American Academy of Pediatrics. (1989). *Report of the committee on infectious diseases* (21st ed.). Elk Grove, IL: Author.

American Academy of Pediatrics. (1990). Children with health impairments in the schools. *Pediatrics, 86*(4), 636-638.

American Academy of Pediatrics. (1991). *Report of the committee on infectious diseases* (22nd ed.). Elk Grove, IL: Author.

American Heart Association & the American Academy of Pediatrics. (1988). *Textbook of pediatric advanced life support.* Dallas, TX : Author.

American Medical Association. (1986). Standards for Cardiopulmonary Resuscitation (CPR) and Emergency Cardiac Care (ECC): Part IV. Pediatric basic life support. *Journal of the American Medical Association, 255*(21), 2954-2960.

Anderson, R. (1988). Management of developmentally disabled children with chronic infections. *Infants and Young Children, 1*(1), 1-9.

Association for the Care of Children's Health. (1989). *Your child with special needs at home and in the community.* Washington, DC: Author.

Bailey, D., Jr. (1991). Issues and perspectives on family assessment. *Infants and Young Children, 4*(1), 26-34.

Batshaw, M., & Perret, Y. (1986). *Children with handicaps: A medical primer* (2nd ed.). Baltimore: Paul H. Brookes.

Benoliel, J. (1975). Childhood diabetes: The commonplace of living becomes uncommon. In A. L. Strauss (Ed.), *Chronic illness and the quality of life* (pp. 89-98). St. Louis: C. V. Mosby.

Blackman, J. (1990). *Medical aspects of developmental disabilities in children birth to three* (2nd ed.). Rockville, MD: Aspen.

Breslau, N., Weitzman, M., & Messenger, K. (1981). Psychological functioning of siblings of disabled children. *Pediatrics, 67*(3), 344-353.

Brewer, E., Jr., McPherson, M., Magrab, P., & Hutchins, V. (1989). Family-centered, community-based, coordinated care for children with special health care needs. *Pediatrics, 83*(6), 1055-1060.

Bricker, D., Bailey, E., & Bruder, M. (1984). The efficacy of early intervention and the handicapped infant: A wise or wasted resource. In M. Wolraich & D. Routh (Eds.), *Advances in developmental and behavioral pediatrics* (pp. 373-423). Greenwich, CT: JAI Press.

Castro, G., & Mastropieri, M. (1986). The efficacy of early intervention: A meta-analysis. *Journal of the Division of Early Childhood, 52*(5), 417-424.

Centers for Disease Control. (1985). *What you can do to stop disease in child care centers.* Atlanta, GA: Department of Health and Human Services.

Centers for Disease Control. (1987). Update: Recommendations for prevention of HIV transmission in health-care settings. *Morbidity and Mortality Weekly Report, 36,* 1-18.

Chasnoff, I., Bussey, M., Savich, R., & Stack, C. (1986). Perinatal cerebral infarction and maternal cocaine use. *Journal of Pediatrics, 108,* 456-459.

Clements, D., Copeland, L., & Loftus, M. (1990). Critical times for families with chronically ill children. *Pediatric Nursing, 16*(2), 157-161.

Cooney, T., & Thurlbeck, W. (1982). Pulmonary hypoplasia in Down syndrome. *New England Journal of Medicine, 307*(19), 1170-1173.

Crowley, A. (1990). Integrating handicapped and chronically ill children into day care centers. *Pediatric Nursing, 16*(1), 39-44.

Dowds, D., & Graham, M. (1989). *Prevention of handicapping conditions in Florida's infants and toddlers: A proposed definition of at-risk.* Tallahassee, FL: Florida Developmental Disabilities Planning Council.

Dunst, C. (1985). Overview of the efficacy of early intervention programs: Methodological and conceptual considerations. In L. Bickman & D. Weatherford (Eds.), *Evaluating early intervention programs for severely handicapped children and their families.* (pp. 79-147). Austin, TX: Pro-Ed.

Dunst, C., Snyder, S., & Mankinen, M. (1986). Efficacy of early intervention. In M. Wang, H. Walber, & M. Reynolds (Eds.), *Handbook of special education: Research and practice, 3,* (pp. 259-294), Oxford, England: Pergaman Press.

Education for the Handicapped Law Report. (1984). Education of the handicapped act and regulations. *Education for the Handicapped Law Report.* Alexandria, VA: CRR Publishing.

Epilepsy Foundation of America. (1985). *Recognizing the hidden signs of childhood seizures.* Landover, MD: Author.

Epilepsy Foundation of America. (1987). *Children and epilepsy: The teacher's role.* Landover, MD: Author.

Epstein, F. (1984). How to keep shunts functioning, or "The impossible dream." *Clinical Neurosurgery, 32,* 608-631.

Esterson, M., & Bluth, L. (1987). *Related services for handicapped children.* Boston: College-Hill Press.

Fox, H., Freedman, S., & Klepper, B. (1989). Financing programs for young children with handicaps. In J. Gallagher, P. Trohanis, & R. Clifford (Eds.), *Policy implementation & P.L. 99-457: Planning for young children with special needs.* (pp 169-182), Baltimore: Paul H. Brookes.

Gallo, A. (1991). Family adaptation in childhood chronic illness: A case report.

Journal of Pediatric Health Care, 5, 78-85.

Graff, J., Ault, M., Guess, D., Taylor, M., & Thompson, B. (1990). *Health care for students with disabilities: An illustrated medical guide for the classroom.* Baltimore: Paul H. Brookes.

Hakes, A. (1990). *Handbook of Florida university programs and standards for professions serving handicapped and at-risk infants, toddlers, and their families: Toward developing a comprehensive system of personnel development required by Public Law 99-457.* Tallahassee, FL: Florida Consortium of Newborn Intervention Programs.

Hanline, M., & Hansen, M. (1989). Integration considerations for infants and toddlers with multiple disabilities. *Journal of the Association for Persons with Severe Handicaps, 14*(3), 178-183.

Harris, R., & Hyman, R. (1984). Clean vs sterile tracheostomy care and level of pulmonary infection. *Nursing Research, 33*(2), 80-85.

Haynes, U. (1983). *Holistic health care for children with developmental disabilities.* Baltimore: University Park Press.

Haynie, M., Porter, S., & Palfrey, J. (1989). *Children assisted by medical technology in education settings: Guidelines for care.* Boston: Project School Care, Children's Hospital.

Holvoet, J., & Helmstetter, E. (1989). *Medical problems of students with special needs: A guide to educators.* Boston: College-Hill Press.

Huddleston, K., & Ferraro, A. (1991). Preparing families of children with gastrostomies. *Pediatric Nursing, 17*(2), 153-158.

Huth, M., & O'Brien, M. (1987). The gastrostomy feeding button. *Pediatric Nursing, 13*(4), 241-245.

Johnson, D. (1991). Grieving is the pits. *Exceptional Parent, 21*(4), 46-48.

Kelley, S., Walsh, J., & Thompson, K. (1991). Birth outcomes, health problems, and neglect with prenatal exposure to cocaine. *Pediatric Nursing, 17*(2), 130-136.

Kennedy, A., Johnson, W., & Sturdevant, E. (1982). An educational program for families of children with tracheostomies. *Maternal Child Nursing, 7*(1), 42-49.

Kohrman, A. (1990). Bringing home a medically complex baby: Psychological issues for families, caretakers, and professionals. *Zero to Three, XI*(2), 36-41.

LeBlanc, P., Parekh, A., Naso, B., & Glass, L. (1987). Effects of intrauterine exposure to alkaloidal cocaine (crack). *American Journal of Diseases in Children, 141,* 937-938.

Levenson, P., & Cooper, M. (1984). School health education for the chronically impaired individual. *Journal of School Health, 54*(11), 446-449.

Levine, B., & Lavi, S. (1991). Perils of childhood immunization against measles, mumps and rubella. *Pediatric Nursing, 17*(2), 159-160, 215.

Lozes, M. (1988). Bladder and bowel management for children with myelomeningocele. *Infants and Young Children, 1*(1), 52-62.

McCubbin, M., & McCubbin, H. (1987). Family stress theory and assessment. In H. I. McCubbin & A. I. Thompson (Eds.), *Family assessment inventories for research and practice* (pp. 3-327). Madison, WI: University of Wisconsin-Madison.

McCubbin, H., & Patterson, J. (1983). Family transitions: Adaptation to stress.

In H. I. McCubbin & C. R. Figley (Eds.), *Stress and the family: Coping with normative transitions (Volume I)* (pp. 5-25). New York: Brunner/Masel.

Monsen, R. (1986). Phases in the caring relationship: From adversary to ally to coordinator. *Maternal Child Nursing, 11*, 316-318.

Morse, M. (1990, Fall). P.L. 94-142 and P.L. 99-457: Considerations for coordination between the health and education systems. *Children's Health Care, 19*(4), 213-218.

Moulton, P. (1984). Chronic illness, grief, and the family. *Journal of Community Health Nursing, 1*(2), 75-88.

Nolan, E. (1991). Infants at risk: A time for action. *Pediatric Nursing, 17*(2), 175-177.

Orelove, F., & Sobsey, D. (1987). *Educating children with multiple disabilities: A transdisciplinary approach.* Baltimore: Paul H. Brookes.

Osbourne, A., Jr. (1984, November). How the courts have interpreted the related services mandate. *Exceptional Children, 51*(3), 249-252.

Perrin, J. (1985). Introduction in N. Hobbs & J. Perrin (Eds.), *Issues in the care of children with a chronic illness* (pp. 1-31). San Francisco: Jossey-Bass.

Persons, C. (1987). *Critical care procedures and protocols: A nursing process approach.* Philadelphia: J. B. Lippincott.

Pinyerd, B. (1983). Siblings of children with myelomeningocele: Examining their perceptions. *Maternal Child Nursing. 12*(1), 61-70.

Rowland, T., Nordstrom, B., Bean, M., & Burkhardt, H. (1981). Chronic upper airway obstruction and pulmonary hypertension in Down syndrome. *American Journal of the Diseases of Children, 135*(11), 1050-1052.

Ruben, R., Newton, J., Jornsay, D., Stein, R., Chambers, H., Liquori, J., & Lawrence, C. (1982). Home care of the pediatric patient with a tracheostomy. *Annals of Otology, Rhinology, & Laryngology, 91*(6), 633-640.

Rustia, J., Hartley, R., Hansen, G., Schulte, D., & Spielman, L. (1984, February). Redefinition of school nursing practice: Integrating the developmentally disabled. *Journal of School Health, 54*(2), 58-62.

Schneider, J., Griffith, D., & Chasnoff, I. (1989). Infants exposed to cocaine in utero: Implications for developmental assessment and intervention. *Infants and Young Children, 2*(1), 25-36.

Segal, G., & Falk, D. (1989). *Shunts.* Chicago, IL: Association for Brain Research.

Sells, C., & Paeth, S. (1987). Health and safety in day care. *Topics in Early Childhood Special Education, 7*(1), 61-72.

Shelton, T., Jeppson, E., & Johnson, B. (1987). *Family-centered care for children with special health care needs.* Washington, DC: Association for the Care of Children's Health and the Bureau of Maternal and Child Health, Public Health Service.

Shonkoff, J., & Hauser-Cram, P. (1987, November). Early intervention for disabled infants and their families: A quantitative analysis. *Pediatrics, 80*(5), 650-658.

Simons, R. (1985). *After the tears.* San Diego, CA: Harcourt Brace Jovanovich.

Steele, S. (1988). Assessing developmental delays in preschool children. *Journal of Pediatric Health Care, 2*(1), 141-145.

Stonestreet, R., Johnston, R., & Acton, S. (1991). Guidelines for real partnerships with parents. *Infant-Toddler Intervention, 1*(1), 37-46.

Talabere, L. (1980). The child with a tracheostomy: A holistic approach to home care. *Topics in Clinical Nursing,* 2(3), 27-44.

Urbano, M. (1987). Family adjustment to the medically complex child. In M. Urbano (Ed), *School health nursing services for medically complex children* (pp. 24-30). Tallahassee, FL: Florida Department of Health and Rehabilitative Services.

Urbano, M. T. (Ed.). (1989). *Children's Medical Services nursing procedure reference guide.* Tallahassee, FL: Florida Department of Health and Rehabilitative Services, Children's Medical Services.

Urbano, M. T. (Ed.). (1989). *Nursing procedure reference guide.* Tallahassee, FL: Department of Health and Rehabilitative Services.

von Windeguth, B., Urbano, M. T., Hayes, J., & Martyn, K. (1988). Analysis of infant risk factors documented by public health nurses. *Public Health Nursing,* 5(3), 165-169.

von Windeguth, B., & Urbano, M. (1989). Cocaine abusing mothers and their infants: A new morbidity brings challenges for nursing care. *Journal of Community Health Nursing,* 6(3), 147-153.

Walker, D. (1984). Care of chronically ill children in the schools. *Pediatric Clinics of North America,* 31(1), 221-233.

Walker, D., Epstein, S., Taylor A., Crocker, A., & Tuttle, G. (1989). *Children's Health Care,* 18(4), 196-201.

Wang, M. (1989). Implementing the state of the art and integration mandates of PL 94-142. In J. J. Gallagher, P. L. Trochanis, & R. Clifford (Eds.). *Policy Implementation & P.L. 99-457* (pp. 33-57). Baltimore: Paul H. Brookes.

Whaley, L., & Wong, D. (1987). *Nursing care of infants and children* (3rd ed.). St. Louis: C. V. Mosby.

Williamson, G. (1987). *Children with spina bifida: Early intervention and preschool programming.* Baltimore: Paul H. Brookes.

Wong, D., & Whaley, L. (1990). *Clinical manual of pediatric nursing* (3rd ed.). St. Louis: C. V. Mosby.

Zechman, R. (1986). *Pediatric adaptive technologies: Gastrostomy tube feeding.* Seattle: University of Washington.

Zelle, R., & Coyner, A. (1983). *Developmentally disabled infants and toddlers: Assessment and intervention.* Philadephia: F. A. Davis.

Ziegler, M. (1989). A parent's perspective: Implementing PL 99-457. In J. J. Gallagher, P. L. Trohanis, & R. M. Clifford (Eds.), *Policy Implementation & P.L. 99-457* (pp.85-94). Baltimore: Paul H. Brookes.

SUBJECT INDEX